AIDS Testing

Gerald Schochetman
J. Richard George
Editors

AIDS Testing
Methodology and Management Issues

Foreword by Walter R. Dowdle

With 38 Illustrations

Springer-Verlag
New York Berlin Heidelberg London Paris
Tokyo Hong Kong Barcelona Budapest

Gerald Schochetman, Ph.D.
Chief,
Laboratory Investigations Branch
Division of HIV/AIDS
National Center for Infectious Diseases
Centers for Disease Control
Atlanta, GA 30333
USA

J. Richard George, Ph.D.
Chief,
Developmental Technology Section
Laboratory Investigations Branch
Division of HIV/AIDS
National Center for Infectious Diseases
Centers for Disease Control
Atlanta, GA 30333
USA

The photograph of microtiter plates used in the cover design was provided by Dr. Gillian Turgeon, Cornell University.

Library of Congress Cataloging-in-Publication Data
AIDS testing: methodology and management issues / Gerald Schochetman, J. Richard George, editors.
p. cm.
Includes bibliographical references and index.
ISBN 0-387-97534-9 (alk. paper)—ISBN 3-540-97534-9 (alk. paper)
1. AIDS (Disease)—Diagnosis. I. Schochetman, Gerald. II. George, J. Richard.
[DNLM: 1. Aquired Immunodeficiency Syndrome—diagnosis. 2. Acquired Immunodeficiency Syndrome—prevention & control. 3. HIV Infections—diagnosis. 4. HIV Infections—prevention & control. WD 308 A288468]
RC607.A26A359 1991
616.97'92075—dc20
DNLM/DLC 91-4852
for Library of Congress

Printed on acid-free paper.

Typeset by Best-set Typesetter Ltd, Hong Kong.
Printed and bound by Edwards Brothers, Inc., Ann Arbor, MI.
Printed in the United States of America.

9 8 7 6 5 4 3 2 1

ISBN 0-387-97534-9 Springer-Verlag New York Berlin Heidelberg
ISBN 3-540-97534-9 Springer-Verlag Berlin Heidelberg New York

Foreword

The human immunodeficiency virus (HIV) infection and aquired immunodeficiency syndrome (AIDS) continue to present a major challenge to health care professionals and society throughout much of the world. In the United States in 1989, HIV/AIDS became the second leading cause of death among men 25 to 44 years of age and ranked eighth among causes of death in women 25 to 44 years of age. On the basis of current trends, HIV/AIDS is expected to rank fifth among the causes of death in women in this age group in 1991.

Testing for the AIDS virus has become a cornerstone for surveillance and prevention programs and for provision of appropriate medical care for those who are infected. Current HIV tests are highly accurate. They rank among the best diagnostic tests in use today. The controversy surrounding the tests now stems not from a lack of confidence in their reliability but from the perceived social consequences of an individual being identified as infected with the AIDS virus. With better understanding by the public of HIV infection/AIDS and a greater acceptance of those who are infected, this attitude can be hoped to change.

The public and private health care sectors have an obligation to those who are infected by HIV and those who are at risk of infection. For health care providers who must understand and apply testing for detection, counseling, and care of HIV-infected persons, this book provides a comprehensive overview of the spectrum of issues relating to HIV testing. Available tests are discussed in terms of information that they provide and the application of that information for the benefit of the patient. Other chapters provide guidance for clinical laboratorians on the design and safe implementation of quality HIV testing procedures.

This book describes in clear terms all the complex elements of testing, including (i) those who should be offered the tests, (ii) medical and ethical considerations, (iii) the scientific principles of the tests, and (iv) application of the tests to determine immune functions and progress of virus infection.

Testing for HIV is an integral component of disease control, even more so as potential vaccines and new therapies are developed. Remarkable progress has been made in the area of HIV testing. Most recent is the application of the polymerase chain reaction (PCR) to detect HIV infection and to trace transmission and evolution of the virus. New tests and new procedures undoubtedly will be developed as more is learned about HIV infection and the opportunities for intervention expand, but this book should remain a valuable reference source for years to come.

Walter R. Dowdle
Deputy Director
Centers for Disease Control

Contents

Contributors

Kenneth G. Castro, M.D., Epidemiology Branch, Division of HIV/AIDS, National Center for Infectious Diseases, Centers for Disease Control, Atlanta, GA 30333

J. Richard George, Ph.D., Chief, Developmental Technology Section, Laboratory Investigations Branch, Division of HIV/AIDS, National Center for Infectious Diseases, Centers for Disease Control, Atlanta, GA 30333

C. Robert Horsburgh, Jr. M.D., Epidemiology Branch, Division of HIV/AIDS, National Center for Infectious Diseases, Centers for Disease Control, Atlanta, GA 30333

M.E. Kennedy, Chief, Office of Biosafety, Laboratory Center for Disease Control, Health and Welfare Canada, Tunney's Pasture, Ottawa, Ontario, Canada, K1A 0L2

Michael D. Lairmore, D.V.M., Ph.D., Department of Veterinary Pathobiology, The Ohio State University, Columbus, OH 43210

Renu Lal, Ph.D., Retrovirus Diseases Branch, Division of Viral and Rickettsial Diseases, National Center for Infectious Diseases, Centers for Disease Control, Atlanta, GA 30333

Alan L. Landay, Ph.D., Director, Immunology Laboratory, Office of Consolidated Laboratory Services, Rush-Presbyterian-St. Luke's Medical Center, Chicago, IL 60612

Alison C. Mawle, Ph.D., Division of HIV/AIDS, National Center for Infectious Diseases, Centers for Disease Control, Atlanta, GA 30333

J. Steven McDougal, M.D., Chief, Immunology Branch, Division of HIV/AIDS, National Center for Infectious Diseases, Centers for Disease Control, Atlanta, GA 30333

Betsy M. Ohlsson-Wilhelm, Ph.D., Departments of Medicine and Microbiology and Immunology, The Pennsylvania State University, College of Medicine, Hershey, PA 17033

Jacquelyn A. Polder, B.S.N., M.P.H., AIDS Activity, Hospital Infections Program, National Center for Infectious Diseases, Centers for Disease Control, Atlanta, GA 30333

Mark A. Rayfield, Ph.D., Chief, Cell Biology Section, Laboratory Investigations Branch, Division of HIV/AIDS, National Center for Infectious Diseases, Centers for Disease Control, Atlanta, GA 30333

Martha F. Rogers, M.D., Chief, Epidemiology Branch, Division of HIV/AIDS, National Center for Infectious Diseases, Centers for Disease Control, Atlanta, GA 30333

Gerald Schochetman, Ph.D., Chief, Laboratory Investigations Branch, Division of HIV/AIDS, National Center for Infectious Diseases, Centers for Disease Control, Atlanta, GA 30333

John J. Sninsky, Ph.D., PCR Division, Cetus Corp., Emoryville, CA 94608

John W. Ward, M.D., Chief, Reporting and Analysis Section, Surveillance Branch, Division of HIV/AIDS, National Center for Infectious Diseases, Centers for Disease Control, Atlanta, GA 30333

1 Testing for AIDS and Human Retroviruses: An Overview

GERALD SCHOCHETMAN

Since the first cases of acquired imunodeficiency syndrome (AIDS) were described in 1981, the global impact of this new epidemic has been dramatic. By December 1990, more than 150 countries had reported over 307,000 cases to the World Health Organization (WHO), and over 8 million persons worldwide were estimated to be infected with the human immunodeficiency virus type 1 (HIV-1), the etiologic agent of AIDS. There are estimated to be at least 1 million HIV-infected persons in the United States alone. Most of these infected persons are expected to develop AIDS. HIV infection throughout the world has continued to be limited to four major modes of transmission: (i) sexual intercourse (vaginal or anal); (ii) transfusion of HIV-contaminated blood or blood products; (iii) sharing of contaminated injection equipment (mainly involved in illegal intravenous drug use); and (iv) transmission from an infected woman to her fetus or infant (perinatal transmission).

HIV-1 was discovered in 1983–1984 and subsequently characterized and shown to belong to a group of viruses known as the lentiviruses, which are a subgroup of the retrovirus family of viruses. It was observed early in the AIDs epidemic that the T4-helper lymphocyte showed a dramatic decline in infected patients. It was subsequently shown that the T4 cells were the principal target of HIV-1 and that their loss was caused by their preferential infection and destruction by the virus. The preferential infection of T4 cells by HIV-1 resulted from the presence of the CD4 protein on the surface of these cells. It was later discovered that monocytes and macrophages, which also express the CD4 protein, could also be infected and become functionally compromised.

Because HIV-1 can integrate its genetic information into the chromosomes of the infected cells, it can remain for the life of the infected cell. The virus can remain in the cell in a quiescent or latent state, or it can become activated through mechanisms as yet unclear, leading to production and spread of the virus. The viral genetic information (in the form of DNA) can replicate with the host's cellular DNA, yielding HIV-infected progeny cells. This ability of HIV results in a lifelong persistent infection of the host and leads to the development of AIDS.

Virus isolation in mitogen-stimulated lymphocytes and successful adaption to growth in continuous T-cell lines made possible the development of tests to detect antibodies to the virus in infected persons. This led to the ability to identify both symptomatic and asymptomatic carriers of the virus. The first commercial tests in the United States, enzyme immunoassays (EIA), were licensed by the Food and Drug Administration (FDA) in 1985 and were immediately used for donated blood and plasma screening. The FDA also approved the licensed EIAs for general diagnostic use as their supply increased. Because any screening test can result in a false-positive reaction, it is necessary to validate positive results by supplemental testing. This has generally been accomplished using mainly Western immunoblots (WB) or, to a lesser extent, the indirect immunofluorescence assay (IFA).

Tests for HIV have been used for three main purposes, namely screening, diagnosis, and surveillance. Efforts to screen for HIV infection have depended primarily on the EIA because it is highly sensitive and specific and because the EIA format is well suited for mass testing. Although initially developed to screen blood donors, the tests have also been used to screen many other groups, including hospitalized patients, military recruits and personnel, prisoners, applicants for marriage licenses, applicants for health and life insurance, childbearing women and their newborns, and immigrants.

Medical diagnostic testing includes detection of HIV infection and staging and prognosis of HIV disease. Antibody screening by EIA, followed by confirmation using WB or IFA, remains the most widely used method of determining HIV infection. However, diagnosis of infection cannot always be based on antibody tests. Antibodies are not present very early in the infection and may be lost in advanced AIDS. Patients with congenital infections or immune deficiencies may not seroconvert (develop detectable virus-specific antibodies). Antibodies can be also passively acquired, as occurs for maternal antibodies in neonates born to HIV-seropositive mothers, although only a small percentage of the neonates are truly infected. In these situations, use has been made of other approaches to determine HIV infection, including direct detection of the virus or its components by culture, analyzing plasma or serum for circulating viral antigen, and the polymerase chain reaction (PCR) technique for viral genetic information. In addition, for perinatal diagnosis, use has been made of assays for cell-surface HIV antibody expression (ELISPOT test) or in vitro HIV antibody production by the patient's lymphocytes.

Surveillance for HIV infection has become a public health priority, to monitor the epidemic and project its future course and impact on society. Once again, the EIA and the WB test for HIV antibodies have been the major analytical tools. Testing of neonatal samples collected as blood spots (collected routinely as part of testing for congenital metabolic disorders) for HIV antibodies has emerged as a useful way to survey infections in childbearing women, an index of horizontal and projected vertical spread of the epidemic.

Progress in HIV testing has been extremely rapid since the discovery of the virus, and the quality of available diagnostic tests rivals that in any other branch of medicine. Nevertheless, improvements are still needed in HIV antibody test sensitivity, specificity, and reproducibility. Antibody tests remain highly practical and will continue to be adapted to the needs in different settings. For purposes of disease staging, more accurate methods are needed to quantitate the virus burden both in the circulation and in target tissues; it is hoped we can correlate the level of virus expression with clinical progression and infectivity. It appears that techniques such as the PCR will help to fulfill this need. Eventually, methods will be needed to distinguish true infection from the presence of antibodies from vaccination or passive immunotherapy. The search for accurate clinically predictive markers remains complex, but is a matter of high priority. Reduction in the cost of HIV testing would be expected to improve the availability of testing worldwide and contribute substantially to disease prevention.

Since the introduction of the first licensed HIV test, the number of tests performed and the number of laboratories performing HIV tests have substantially increased. However, programs to quality control laboratory testing have barely kept pace. With the prospect of even more testing in the future, there will be an increasing need for laboratories to develop and implement appropriate quality control programs to ensure reliable testing.

Progress in prognostic testing has been hampered by the limited understanding of the relationships among virus expression, immune responses, and clinical manifestations. The number of circulating T4-helper cells (the main target of HIV infection) has been the most consistent correlate of clinical progression. However, independent prognostic value has also been shown for detectable p24 antigen, decrease in titer of anti-p24, and elevated values of beta-2 microglobulin and neopterin. Clinical progression also correlates with an increase in the titer of infectious virus in both plasma (viremia) and circulating lymphocytes (infected cell burden). The development of sensitive and specific predictive laboratory markers for disease progression in HIV infection is critical in accelerating the development of antiviral drugs, because drug trials must otherwise depend on clinical endpoints which may take years to reach.

A second AIDS virus, HIV-2, was discovered in 1986 and shown to be endemic in parts of West Africa with limited spread mainly in Western Europe. In the United States, approximately 24 cases of HIV-2 infection have been documented, and surveillance studies confirm a very low prevalence of infection in the United States and Canada. Serologic tests for HIV-2 have been developed that are similar to those developed for HIV-1. Combination tests for HIV-1 and HIV-2 are currently being used to screen donated blood in parts of Europe where the prevalence of HIV-2 infection warrants intervention. Because of the low prevalence of HIV-2 in the United States, the FDA has concluded that blood donor screening for HIV-2 antibodies does not appear to be necessary at this time. In contrast, because of increased concern about transmission of human T-cell leukemia/lymphoma virus (HTLV) -I and HTLV-II through blood transfusion, screening and diagnostic tests for antibodies to these agents have been developed and implemented for screening donated blood. HTLV-1, the first human retrovirus described, is a transforming virus known to cause a highly malignant cancer termed adult T-cell leukemia/lymphoma (ATL) and a demylinating disease known as tropical spastic parparesis (TSP) or HTLV-I-associated myelopathy (HAM). Shortly after the discovery of HTLV-I, a closely related retrovirus, HTLV-II, was isolated from two patients with a rare form of leukemia known as hairy cell leukemia.

Counseling has been a crucial adjunct to HIV testing, both in regard to effecting and enhancing behavioral change and in referring HIV-seropositive persons for medical evaluation and treatment. The role of testing and counseling in behavior change has been studied extensively in homosexual men. The wider relevance of HIV counseling and testing conclusions in other settings will require additional evaluation. Sound medical indications and goals that benefit both the public health and the health of the individual must be the basis of HIV counseling and testing. The goal of testing and counseling is to encourage more people to seek HIV testing services to reduce the rate of HIV transmission and associated HIV illnesses. To achieve this, testing should be performed by an experienced laboratory in a supportive environment with proper consent and confidentiality policies. The individual being tested should also receive effective prevention messages coupled with proper medical referral.

Biosafety guidelines have been published to reduce the risk of HIV infection among workers who might be exposed to the virus while performing their job duties. The universal infection control precautions outlined in these guidelines remain the primary means of preventing occupational HIV infection, and these safety guidelines should be strictly followed. Additional recommendations have been suggested for management of workers following occupational exposure to HIV-infected material. These include emergency treatment immediately after an exposure, initial and follow-up testing to monitor for seroconversion and infection, and the use of zidovudine for postexposure prophylaxis to potentially prevent HIV infection.

The AIDS virus (and other human retroviruses) will be with us for quite some time. There is much yet to learn about this virus and the AIDS pandemic that it has spawned. This book is a beginning in presenting a clear and comprehensive picture concerning HIV testing and the numerous issues associated with it.

2 Testing for Human Retroviral Infections: Medical Indications and Ethical Considerations

JOHN W. WARD

In 1985, the first tests became available to identify antibody to a retrovirus, the human immunodeficiency virus (HIV). Since that time, HIV antibody testing has become the cornerstone of public health efforts to stop the epidemic of HIV infection. The tests were used initially to screen donated blood and plasma, and their use for this purpose dramatically decreased the rate of transfusion-associated HIV transmission.[1,2] Soon thereafter, testing linked with counseling was recommended as a method to encourage safer sexual and drug use practices[3,4] and to aid in the diagnosis of some conditions included in the acquired immunodeficiency syndrome (AIDS).[5]

The major benefits of HIV testing are counseling to promote the behavior change necessary to reduce HIV transmission and the referral of HIV-seropositive persons for medical evaluation and treatment. As part of counseling, information is provided to persons who seek testing regarding the modes of HIV transmission and how the risk of transmission can be reduced. This information frequently results in these persons changing high-risk sexual or drug use behaviors to prevent HIV infection in themselves and others.[6–10] Also, women at risk for infection receive information regarding perinatal transmission of HIV, and women found HIV seropositive may elect to avoid pregnancy. Although counseling can be performed in the absence of HIV testing, knowledge of HIV seropositivity may be an additional motivator for behavior change.[6–8]

The development of new medical therapies for HIV infection and associated illnesses have strengthened the medical indications for testing. In the summer of 1989, the early use of zidovudine was found to delay the progression to AIDS for HIV-infected individuals.[11] Other prophylactic and therapeutic regimens such as aerosolized pentamidine for *Pneumocystis carinii* pneumonia, chemotherapy for tuberculosis, and pneumococcal vaccination may delay or prevent HIV-associated conditions.[11–14] These findings are expected to significantly increase the number of persons seeking to learn their HIV serologic status. Of the approximately 1 million HIV-infected persons, an estimated 460,000–675,000 have sufficient immunodeficiency to warrant medical therapy by the most recent treatment guidelines.[15]

As the uses of the tests have expanded, there has been a concomitant increase in concerns regarding the indications for testing and the possible adverse consequences for individuals testing positive for HIV infection.[16–19] There was initial concern about the reliability of the tests and the meaning of a positive test result. Subsequent studies of test performance have shown the HIV antibody tests to be both highly sensitive and specific and that a positive antibody (Ab) test almost invariably indicates a current HIV infection.[20–23] However, false-positive test results remain a possibility and may cause persons to receive incorrect test information.[24] The laboratory reporting of test results to the clinician may also be erroneous or vague.[25,26] Although these instances of poor reporting are probably uncommon, such instances may result in unnecessary anxiety and changes in career and family planning.[27]

Protection from discrimination is particularly important for HIV testing as the populations at greatest risk for HIV infection—homosexual and bisexual men, intravenous drug users, and racial and ethnic minorities—are already prone to discrimination by society. Individuals known to be infected with HIV have experienced a loss of employment, housing, and health or life insurance.[28,29] Health care workers may also refuse to care for HIV-seropositive persons.[23,24] In addition, HIV-seropositive persons are asked to inform their sexual partners, which may result in the destruction of marriages and other personal relationships.[30]

To maximize the benefits and reduce the risk of HIV antibody testing, the Public Health Service and other authorities have reviewed the medical and ethical issues regarding HIV testing and have recommended certain practices and procedures.[3,4,27,30–32] To benefit the individual tested, testing should have the proper medical indications and should be linked with counseling and referral for appropriate evaluations and treatment. To increase the safety of the test procedure, HIV testing is recommended to be voluntary, with informed consent and with procedures to protect the confidentiality of test results.[33]

This chapter primarily addresses testing for HIV antibody as this is the most common screening test for HIV infection. However, the efforts to maximize benefits of testing and minimize risks for tested individuals also apply to other tests for HIV infection and for other retroviral testing such as for human T-lymphotropic virus (HTLV) type I/II.

Indications for Testing

Not everyone needs HIV antibody testing. Knowledge of the behaviors that place persons at risk for HIV infection and of the clinical conditions associated with HIV infection is required to properly target HIV counseling and testing to those most in need of these services. Testing persons who are not at risk for HIV infection unnecessarily lowers the predictive value of a positive test and needlessly adds to the cost of public health programs and medical care. Persons who should be offered HIV counseling and testing include the following:

Persons with Behavioral Risks for HIV Infection

Persons at risk for HIV infection include homosexual/bisexual men, present or past intravenous drug users, male or female prostitutes, sex partners of infected persons or persons at increased risk, all persons with hemophilia who received clotting factor concentrate before 1985, and newborn infants of mothers with risks for HIV infection.[4] To identify risks associated with HIV transmission, physicians and other health care providers should interview patients regarding their sexual and drug use practices and their transfusion history. HIV counseling and testing should be recommended for persons who self-report risks or for whom risks for HIV infection have been identified.

Conditions Associated with HIV Infection

The test is a useful diagnostic tool for evaluating patients with clinical or laboratory evidence of HIV infection. Since 1987, the Centers for Disease Control (CDC) have allowed a diagnosis of certain conditions indicative of underlying immunosuppression if persons are positive for HIV antibody.[5] Also, some medical conditions are found more often among persons infected with HIV, including pneumonia caused by *Streptococcus pneumonia* or *Haemophilus influenza*.[34] In addition, *Mycobacterium* tuberculosis infection is recognized as an HIV-associated condition. All persons with tuberculosis should be offered counseling and testing for HIV infection.[14,35]

Recipients of Transfusions Between 1978 and 1985

Persons who received transfusions of blood or blood components during this time period are at the greatest risk of transfusion-associated (TA) HIV transmission. An estimated 12,000 living persons were infected with HIV before HIV testing of blood donors was initiated.[36] The risk of TA transmission is greatest for persons who received relatively large numbers of units in areas of the countries with high rates of AIDS and HIV infection.[36]

A priority for HIV prevention efforts is to provide access to counseling and testing for persons who are most likely to be infected with HIV. Persons with certain clinical conditions are at increased risk of HIV infection:

Persons with Other Sexually Transmitted Diseases

All persons seeking treatment for a sexually transmitted disease (STD) should be routinely offered HIV-related counseling and testing.[4] HIV testing is particularly important for persons with other STDs as they may not otherwise recognize their risk for HIV infection. Persons with STDs are practicing behaviors that may also transmit HIV and may have significant rates of HIV infection. Since 1988, CDC has conducted an HIV seroprevalence study of anonymous specimens from persons seeking treatment in STD clinics.[33] Of 115,989 clients seen in 85 clinics in 31 metropolitan areas, a median of 2.5% (range, 0–39%) were HIV seropositive.[34]

Persons Receiving Treatment for Intravenous Drug Use

Intravenous drug use is a behavior at high risk for HIV transmission, and persons in drug treatment programs have high rates of HIV infection. Of the 15,000 intravenous drug users in 27 metropolitan areas who tested as part of the CDC blinded seroprevalence study,[38] 5.0% were HIV seropositive (range, 0–47%).[36] Although the rate of HIV infection is higher in the Northeast (median, 18.2%) than in the rest of the United States (median, 2.5%) all intravenous drug users can benefit from counseling and testing to promote safer behavior and reduce further HIV transmission. Previous prevention efforts targeted to intravenous drug users have shown success in decreasing high-risk needle-sharing practices but less improvement in reducing the frequency of high-risk sexual activity.[6]

Women of Reproductive Age

Women at risk for HIV infection should be offered counseling and testing services. Women at risk include those who have used intravenous drugs, have engaged in prostitution, have received a transfusion of blood in the period 1978–1985, have had sexual partners who are infected with HIV or who are at risk for HIV infection, and women who live in communities where there is a known or suspected high prevalence of HIV infection.[4]

Although the HIV seroprevalence among women is low, women benefit from testing as they may be more likely than men to be unaware of their risk for HIV infection.[40] Offering HIV testing to all women in areas with high HIV seroprevalence is particularly important because many women may not report a risk for HIV infection on interview.[41] In a CDC survey of 100,000 women of reproductive age in 32 metropolitan areas,[42] the median rate of HIV infection was 0.2% (range, 0–2.3%) with the median seroprevalence rate among black women (0.5%; range, 0–3.5%) greater than among white (0%; range, 0–4.3%) and Hispanic women (0%; 0–2.5%).[43]

In addition, the availability of HIV testing and counseling for women is one prevention strategy to reduce the risk of perinatal HIV transmission. The offering of HIV counseling and testing allows women of childbearing age to determine their serologic status and to become aware of the risk of perinatal HIV transmission. These women may then decide whether they wish to delay becoming pregnant or to continue current pregnancies. To identify the rate in childbearing women, CDC has conducted a study in 24 states testing anonymous specimens collected from newborns for maternal HIV antibody.[44] The HIV seroprevalence rate was 0.15% in the childbearing women tested; if this rate is projected nationally, an estimated 1,500–2,000 children are infected annually by perinatal HIV transmission.

General Hospital Admissions in Some Areas

The rate of HIV seroprevalence among persons admitted to hospitals in some areas is high.[45–50] Preliminary data from a CDC sentinel hospital network are available from 26 sentinel hospitals in 21 cities for the period from January 1988 through June 1989.[47] Specimens collected from a sample of patients are stripped of personal identifiers and are excluded if the patient has an admitting diagnosis of AIDS or HIV-related conditions, or has other medical conditions likely to be associated with HIV. Of 89,547 blood specimens tested, 1,201 (1.3%) were positive for HIV antibody. The seroprevalence rate among the participating hospitals ranged from 0.1% to 7.8%. Hospitals with high rates of HIV infections tend to be in areas of the country with high rates of HIV infection and AIDS.

Based on these and other data,[36–50] all hospitals and their associated providers should consider whether HIV counseling and testing services should be routinely offered to all or selected patients receiving care in their facilities. Hospitals may elect to target HIV testing to persons 18–44 years of age because 92% of the infected persons identified in the CDC sentinel hospital study were in this age range.

Persons with Tuberculosis

All persons with tubercular infection or tuberculosis need to be assessed for HIV infection.[14,35] *Mycobacterium tuberculosis* infection is frequently found among HIV-infected persons. Approximately 4% of persons with AIDS in 43 states and 11 localities have been reported as having tuberculosis.[35] In San Francisco and Seattle, the rate of HIV infection among persons with tuberculosis is 29% and 23%, respectively.[51,52] Coinfection with HIV and *M.* tuberculosis may cause tuberculosis to develop more quickly and to precede the development of AIDS. In a cohort of methadone maintenance clients with positive tuberculin skin test reactions, 14% of the HIV-infected persons as compared to none (0%) of the HIV-seronegative clients developed tuberculosis during a 2-year follow-up period.[53] In Florida, 62 (57%) of 109 AIDS patients with tuberculosis had developed tuberculosis 1 month or more before their diagnosis of AIDS.[54] Thus, latent subclinical tuberculous infection may often progress to clinical tuberculosis early in the course of HIV-related immunosuppression.

Persons with positive tuberculin skin test reactions should be interviewed regarding their risk for HIV infection and HIV counseling, and testing should be strongly encouraged if risks are identified. Persons with tuberculosis or positive skin test reactions should be given or referred for the appropriate therapy.[14,35]

Guidelines for HIV Counseling and Testing

The proper counseling and testing procedures are important to maximize the benefits and reduce the risks of HIV testing. More people will seek HIV testing if they are confident about the testing program and can recognize the benefits of testing for themselves. The following recommendations were developed to standardize the methods of providing HIV counseling and testing services provided for persons in the acute clinical care setting.

Laboratory Testing and Reporting

Laboratories that perform HIV testing should be familiar with HIV test procedures and should use standardized criteria for test interpretation.[25] The HIV counseling process begins with reporting the test results. Thus, laboratory reports should contain clear language describing what test were performed and their interpretation.[26] HIV test results should be recorded on the medical record, and every effort should be used to ensure the confidentiality of test results. A careful review of record-keeping practices and how medical information is maintained and distributed can help to identify ways to stop the unnecessary disclosure of patient information. Except for reporting of test results to local and state health departments where required, test results should not be distributed to individuals or institutions outside the hospital or testing center without consent of the tested individual.

Informed Consent

Testing for HIV infection should be voluntary and persons should be able to refuse testing. Mandatory HIV testing is not recommended as a method to prevent most HIV transmission. The public health uses of mandatory testing are primarily limited to the screening of organ, plasma, blood, and other tissue donors. The testing of patients to prevent the risk of occupational HIV transmission has not been shown to be effective. In one study, the frequency of parenteral or cutaneous contact was not influenced by a health care worker's knowledge of the patient's HIV seropositivity or behavioral risks for HIV infection.[26] Prevention efforts continue to depend on persons receiving prevention messages and voluntarily changing high-risk behaviors. Persons must seek or agree to HIV testing voluntarily to initiate the process of voluntary behavior change.

Specific informed consent is required for HIV testing. The informed consent for HIV testing should be separate from the general consent for other medical services.[31,32] Before testing, the patient should be informed why the tests are being performed, what are the benefits and risks of testing, and how the test results will be protected from disclosure.

HIV-Related Counseling Services

HIV-related counseling services should be provided to persons before and after testing. Persons who conduct counseling should have a good working knowledge of HIV infection and should be able to explain ways to modify unsafe sexual and drug use practices. For persons found HIV seropositive, counselors should be able to provide or arrange for appropriate medical evaluation, and if necessary, notification of sexual or needle-sharing partners.

Pretest Counseling

Pretest counseling should consist of information about the procedures of the testing program, the risks for HIV infection, and the meaning of a positive and negative test.[33] Pretest counseling should also include an assessment of the patient's risk for HIV infection and ways to reduce that risk. Persons who report intravenous drug use should be advised to discontinue drug use or, if they cannot do so, to avoid sharing needles and other injection equipment with other persons. If sharing of needles and other equipment continues, the equipment should be washed with bleach before use. Persons with multiple sexual partners should be informed that sexual abstinence or avoiding sexual partners not known to be uninfected with HIV are the optimal ways to eliminate the risk of sexual transmission of HIV. Otherwise, condoms should be used during sexual contact. The risk of perinatal transmission should be discussed with women and with men with female sexual contacts.

Posttest Counseling

After testing, patients should be informed of their test results. HIV-seronegative persons should be informed that a negative test result does not indicate protection from acquiring HIV infection and that continued high-risk sexual or drug use behaviors could result in HIV infection. These persons should also be advised that HIV antibody tests may not detect infection that occurred in the several weeks or months immediately before testing. Persons concerned about a recent exposure should be advised to seek repeated testing at least 6 months after the exposure.

HIV-seropositive patients should be counseled by persons who are able to interpret the test results correctly and who can discuss the medical, social, and psychological implications of HIV infection.[28] A reassessment of a patient's risk for infection is also helpful to focus risk reduction messages and to evaluate the validity of test results. Repeat HIV testing may be necessary for HIV-seropositive persons without identified risk factors.[27] Accurate counseling helps infected persons avoid behaviors that may transmit HIV and helps them to cope with the test information. Counseling should convey some hope and cautious optimism. It is not known if all HIV-infected persons will develop AIDS, and therapeutic approaches are increasingly more effective in delaying or preventing HIV-related illnesses.[11–14]

Partner Notification

Sexual and needle-sharing partners of HIV-infected persons are also at risk for HIV. Persons who are HIV antibody positive should be instructed how to notify their partners and to refer them for counseling and testing. If the HIV-infected persons are reluctant to notify partners directly, counselors should offer to inform partners or to refer the names of partners to the local health department.[30,33] As a last resort, health care providers may need to exercise their legal and ethical duty to inform known sexual and needle-sharing partners of HIV-infected persons who refuse to inform these persons themselves.[27,28,30,33] When others are notifying partners, the name of the infected person should not be used unless consent is given.

Medical Evaluation

To identify those who may benefit from therapy, a medical evaluation is necessary for persons found to be infected with HIV. Physicians, clinics, or other institutions who offer testing should be able to provide a medical evaluation or have an effective referral system for these services. The medical evaluation of HIV-infected persons should include a physical examination, complete blood count with differential, lymphocyte subset analysis, syphilis serology, and a purified protein derivative skin test for tuberculosis.[33] Following evaluation, persons should be referred for the appropriate medical therapy.

In summary, HIV counseling and testing must be based on sound medical indications and have goals that benefit the public health and the health of the individual. The benefits of testing are greatest when persons are tested by a reliable and experienced laboratory in a supportive atmosphere with proper consent and confidentiality procedures, and then receive effective prevention messages and appropriate medical referral services. Access to HIV testing programs with these characteristics will encourage more persons to seek HIV testing services and reduce the rate of HIV transmission and HIV-related illnesses.

References

1. CDC. Provisional Public Health Service inter-agency recommendations for screening donated blood and plasma for antibody to the virus causing acquired immunodeficiency syndrome. MMWR 1985;34:1–5.
2. Ward JW, Holmberg SD, Allen JR, Cohn DL, Critchley SE, Kleinman SH, Lenes BA, Ravenholt O, Davis JR, Quinn MG, Jaffe HW. Human immunodeficiency virus (HIV) transmission by blood transfusions screened negative for HIV antibody. N Engl J Med 1988;318:473–478.
3. CDC. Additional recommendations to reduce sexual and drug abuse related transmission of human T-lymphotropic virus type III/lymphadenopathy-associated virus. MMWR 1986;35:152–155.
4. CDC. Public health service guidelines for counseling and antibody testing to prevent HIV infection and AIDS. MMWR 1987;36:509–515.
5. CDC. Revision of the CDC surveillance case definition for acquired immunodeficiency syndrome. MMWR 1987;36:1–15S.
6. DesJarlais DC, Friedman SR. The psychology of preventing AIDS among intravenous drug users: a social learning conceptualization. Am Psychol 1988; 43:865–70.
7. Godfried JP, Van Griensven MS, Ernest MM, De Vroome MS, Tielman RAP, Goudsmit J, et al. Impact of HIV antibody testing on changes in sexual behavior among homosexual men in the Netherlands. Am J Public Health 1988;78:1575–1577.
8. McCusker J, Stoddard AM, Mayer KH, Zapka JG, Morrussen C, Saltzman MS. Effect of HIV antibody test knowledge on subsequent sex behaviors in a cohort of homosexual men. Am J Public Health 1988; 78:462–467.
9. McCusker J, Stoddard AM, Zapka JG, Zorn M, Mayer KH. Predictors of AIDS preventive behavior among homosexually active men: a longitudinal study. AIDS 1989;3:443–448.
10. Schechter MT, Craib KJ Willoughby B, Douglas B, McLeod WA, Maynard M, et al. Patterns of sexual behavior and condom use in a cohort of homosexual men. Am J Public Health 1988;78:1535–1538.
11. Volberding PA, Lagakos SW, Koch MA, Pettinelli C, Myers MW, Booth DK, Balfour HH, Reichmaor RL, Bartlett JA, Hirsch MS, Murphy RL, Hardy D, Soeiro R, Fischl MA, Bartlett JG, Merigar TC, Hyslop NE, Reichmeor DD, Vakortine FT, Corey L, on the AIDS Clinical Trick Group of the National Institute of Allergy and Infectious Diseases. Zidovudine in

asymptomatic human immunodeficiency virus infection. N Engl J Med 1990; 322:941–949.
12. CDC. Guidelines for prophylaxis against *Pneumocystis carinii* pneumonia for persons infected with human immunodeficiency virus disease. MMWR 1989; 38:Suppl. S5.
13. CDC. General recommendations on immunization. MMWR 1989;38:207–227.
14. CDC. Screening for tuberculosis and tuberculous infection in high-risk populations and the use of preventive therapy for tuberculous infection in the United States. Recommendations of the advisory committee for elimination of tuberculosis. MMWR 1990;39:RR-8.
15. CDC. Estimates of HIV prevalence and projected AIDS cases: summary of a workshop, October 31–November 1, 1989. MMWR 1990;39:110–112, 117–119.
16. Henry K, Maki M, Crossley K. Analysis of the use of HIV antibody testing in a Minnesota hospital. JAMA 1986;259:229–232.
17. Sherer R. Physician use of the HIV antibody test: the need for consent, counseling, confidfentiality, and caution. JAMA 1988;259:264–265.
18. Dickens BM. Legal rights and duties in the AIDS epidemic. Science 1988; 239:580.
19. Walters L. Ethical issues in the prevention and treatment of HIV infection and AIDS. Science 1988;239:597.
20. Ward JW, Grindon AJ, Feorino PM, Schable C, Parvin M., Allen JR. Laboratory and epidemiologic evaluation of an enzyme immunoassay for antibodies to HTLV-III. JAMA 1986;256:357–361.
21. Weiss SH, Goedart JJ, Sarngadharan MB, Bodner AJ, the AIDS seroepidemiology collaborative working group, Gallo RC, Blattner WA. Screening test for HTLV-III (AIDS) agent antibodies: specificity, sensitivity, and applications. JAMA 1985;253:221–225.
22. CDC. Update: serologic testing for antibody to human immunodeficiency virus. MMWR 1988;36:833–40,845.
23. Ou CY, Kwok S, Mitchell SW, Mack DH, Sninsky JJ, Krebs JW, et al. DNA amplification for direct detection of HIV-1 in DNA of peripheral blood mononuclear cells. Science 1988;239:295–297.
24. Saag MS, Britz J. Asymptomatic blood donor with a false positive HTLV III western blot. N Engl J Med 1986;314:118.
25. CDC. Interpretation and use of the western blot assay for serodiagnosis of human immunodeficiency virus type 1 infections. MMWR 1989;38(Suppl 7S).
26. Benenson AS, Peddercord M, Hofherr LK, Ascher MS, Tayor RN, Hearn TL. Reporting the results of human immunodeficiency virus testing. JAMA 1989;262:3435–3438.
27. Lo B, Steinbrook RL, Cooke M. Coates TJ, Walters EJ, Hulley SB. Voluntary screening for human immunodeficiency virus (HIV) infection. Ann Intern Med 1989;110:727–733.
28. Gostin LO. The AIDS litigation project; a national review of court and human rights commission decisions, Part I: The social impact of AIDS. JAMA 1990;263:1961–1969.
29. Gostin LO. The AIDS litigation project; a national review of court and human rights commission decisions, Part II: Discrimination. JAMA 1990;263: 2086–2093.

30. Landesman SH, DeHovitz JA. HIV diagnostic testing: ethical, legal, and clinical considerations. Sex Transm Dis 1990;81:975–983.
31. Bayer R. Editorial review. Ethical and social policy issues raised by HIV screening: the epidemic evolves and so do the challenges. AIDS 1989;3: 119–124.
32. Levine C, Bayer R. The ethics of screening for early intervention in HIV disease. Am J Public Health 1989;79:1661–1667.
33. CDC. 1989 sexually transmitted diseases treatment guidelines. MMWR 1989; 38:S-8.
34. Pizzo PA, Eddy J, Faloon J. Acquired immune deficiency syndrome in children. Current problems and therapeutic considerations. Am J Med 1988; 85:195–202.
35. CDC. Tuberculosis and human immunodeficiency virus infection: recommendations of the advisory committee for the elimination of tuberculosis (ACET). MMWR 1989;3:236–38, 243–250.
36. CDC. Human immunodeficiency virus infection in transfusion recipients and their family members. MMWR 1987;36:137–140.
37. McCray E, Onorato IM, and state and local health departments. HIV seroprevalence in clients attending sexually transmitted disease (STD) clinics in the United States, 1988–90. In: Abstracts, VIth International Conference on AIDS, San Francisco, F.C.44:1990.
38. Jones TS, Allen DM, Onorato IM, Petersen LR, Dondero TJ, Pappaioanou M. HIV seroprevalence surveys in drug treatment centers. Public Health Rep 1990;105:125–130.
39. Allen DM, Onorato IM, Sweeney FA, and state and local health departments. Seroprevalence of HIV infection in intravenous drug users (IVDUs) in the United States (U.S.). In. VIth International Conference on AIDS, San Francisco, F.C.551:1990.
40. Ward JW, Kleinman SH, Douglas DK Grindon AJ, Holmberg SD. Epidemiologic characteristics of blood donors with antibody to human immunodeficiency virus. Transfusion (Philadelphia) 1983;23:298–301.
41. Lindsay MK, Peterson HB, Feng TI, Slade BA, Willis S, Klein L. Routine antepartum human immunodeficiency virus infection screening in an inner city population. Obstet Gynecol 1989;74:289–294.
42. Allen DM, Lee NC, Schulz SL, Pappaioanou M, Dondero TJ, Onorato IM. Determining HIV seroprevalence among women in women's health clinics. Public Health Rep 1990;105:130–134.
43. Sweeney PA, Allen D, Onorato I, and state and local health departments. HIV seroprevalence among women of reproductive age seeking clinic services, United States, 1988–1990. In: Abstracts, VIth International Conference on AIDS, San Francisco, F.C.568:1990.
44. Gwinn M, Pappaioanou M, George R, Hannon WH, Wasser SL, Redus MA, et al. Prevalence of HIV infection in childbearing women in the United States: Surveillance using newborn blood samples. JAMA 1991;265:1704–1708.
45. St. Louis ME, Rauch KJ, Petersen LR, Anderson JE, Schable CA, Donbro TJ, et al. Seroprevalence rates of human immunodeficiency virus infection at sentinel hospitals in the United States. J Engl J Med. 1990;323:213–8.

46. Kelen GD, DiGiovanna T, Bisson L, Kalainov D, Sivertson KT, Quinn TC. Human immunodeficiency virus infection in emergency department patients. JAMA 1989;262:516–522.
47. Soderstrom CA, Furth PA, Glasser D, Dunning RW, Groseclose SL, Cowley RA. HIV infection rates in a trauma center treating predominantly rural blunt trauma victims. J Trauma 1989;29:1526–1530.
48. Lewandowski C; Ognjan A; Rivers E; Pohlod D, Belian B, Saravolatz LD. HIV-1 and HTLV-I seroprevalence in critically ill resuscitated emergency department patients. In: Abstracts for the Vth International Conference on AIDS. Montreal, Canada: Health and Welfare Canada, 1989:142.
49. Gordin FM, Gibert C, Hawley HP, Willoughby A. Prevalence of human immunodeficiency virus and hepatitis B virus in unselected hospital admissions: Implications for mandatory testing and universal precautions. J Infect Dis 1990;161:14–17.
50. Risi GF, Gaumer RH, Weeks S, Leete JK, Sanders CV. Human Immunodeficiency virus: risk of exposure among health care workers at a southern urban hospital. South Med J 1989;82:1079–1082.
51. Chaisson RE, Theuer CP, Schecter GF, Hopewell PC. HIV infection in patients with tuberculosis (Abstract). In: Abstracts, IVth International Conference on AIDS, Stockholm, Book 2, 1988:313.
52. Holan CM, Heckbert S, Elarth A, Hopkins S. A case-control study of the association between human immunodeficiency virus infection and tuberculosis. In: Abstracts, IVth International Conference on AIDS, Stockholm, Book 2, 1988:216.
53. Selwyn PA, Hartel D, Lewis VA, Schoenbaum EE, Vermund SH, Kleior RS, et al. A prospective study of the risk of tuberculosis among intravenous drug users with human immunodeficiency virus infection. N Engl J Med 1989;320: 545–550.
54. CDC. Tuberculosis and acquired immunodeficiency syndrome—Florida. MMWR 1986;35:587–590.

3
Biology of Human Immunodeficiency Viruses

GERALD SCHOCHETMAN

The etiologic agent of AIDS, the human immunodeficiency virus type 1 (HIV-1), was first isolated in 1983–1984 from patients with AIDS-related complex (ARC) and AIDS.[1-3] HIV-1 is the predominant AIDS virus and is found worldwide, primarily in Central Africa, Europe, and North and South America. A second AIDS virus, HIV-2,[4-6] closely related to the simian immunodeficiency virus (SIV), was discovered in 1986 and shown to be endemic in parts of West Africa with limited spread in Western Europe. HIV-2 is only now beginning to appear in the Americas, mainly in the United States, Canada, and Brazil. Infection with either HIV-1 or HIV-2 results in a number of biological and pathological changes leading to a spectrum of immune dysfunctions, neurologic disorders, and enteropathy and AIDS.

The Retrovirus Family

The human immunodeficiency viruses are members of the retrovirus family of viruses.[7] The retroviruses are so called because at the beginning of their life cycle they reverse the usual flow of genetic information in a cell. In all living organisms and in many other viruses, genetic information is stored as DNA and later transcribed into RNA. By contrast, retroviruses store their genetic information as RNA and also contain a unique enzyme, reverse transcriptase (RT), which catalyzes the reverse transcription of the RNA genome (its entire complement of genes) into a DNA copy. The resulting DNA, termed the provirus, can be perceived by the host cell as its own and is integrated into its chromosomal DNA where the provirus can remain dormant for weeks, months, or even years without being expressed, that is, it remains latent. The integrated state is responsible for the persistent nature of retrovirus infections.

The retrovirus family is composed of three subfamilies: oncoviruses, spumaviruses, and lentiviruses (Table 3.1 and Figure 3.1). The oncoviruses, or cancer-causing viruses, are found to be transmitted horizon-

Table 3.1. Subfamilies of retroviruses.

Subfamily	Examples
Oncoviruses:	Associated with the activation of certain cell genes leading to tumor development
Type A	Mouse intracisternal type A
Type B	Mouse mammary tumor virus
Type C	Murine leukemia virus
	Human T-cell leukemia virus types I and II
	Feline leukemia virus
	Bovine leukemia virus
Type D	Mason–Pfizer virus
	SAIDS virus
Spumavirus:	Readily isolated from humans and other primates, but have not been associated with any specific disease
	Simian foamy virus
	Human foamy virus
Lentiviruses:	Produce acute cytocidal infection followed by a slowly developing multisystem disease
	Visna maedi virus
	Caprine arthritis encephalitis virus
	Equine infectious anemia virus
	Feline immunodeficiency virus
	Bovine immunodeficiency virus
	Simian immunodeficiency virus
	Human immunodeficiency virus type 1 (HIV-1) and type 2 (HIV-2)

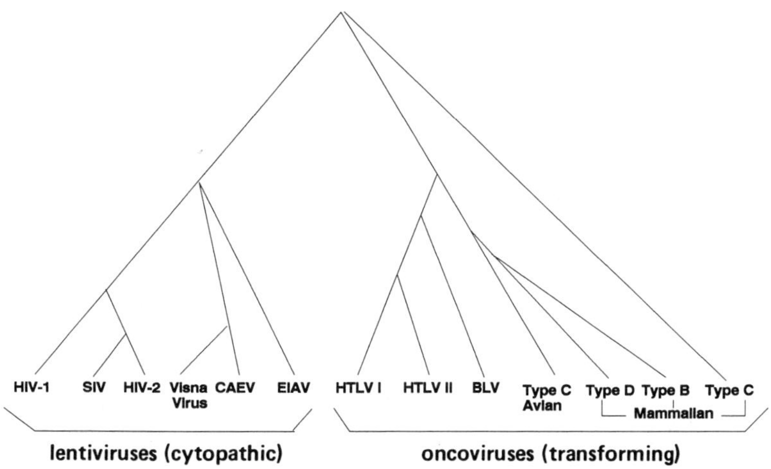

Figure 3.1. Evolutionary relationships of retroviruses.

tally by host-to-host contact and vertically as integrated viruses in germ cells. When integrated into the host DNA, oncoviruses efficiently transform the host cells that have a tumor-producing potential. The lentiviruses and the spumaviruses (spuma for foamy) do not cause cancer and do not integrate into the host's germ cell lines; that is, there is no genetic transmission through the maternal or paternal germ line. Both the lentiviruses and the spumaviruses produce a persistent lifelong infection of the host cells. However, of the two only the lentiviruses have been identified as causes of human and animal diseases. Classification of HIV as a lentivirus is based on its fine structure, biological properties, and protein and nucleic acid sequence homology (Table 3.2). As with other lentiviruses, mature extracellular particles of HIV are characteristically 90–130 nm in diameter and have a double-membraned envelope surrounding an electron-dense cylindrically shaped core.

Relationship of HIV-1 to HIV-2

The genetic similarity between HIV-1 and HIV-2[8,9] is significantly less (40–50% nucleotide identity) than is found among different HIV-1 isolates (greater than 85% nucleotide identity). However, serologic cross-reactive antibodies, mainly to the *gag* and *pol* proteins, from patients infected with either virus can be detected using commercially available serologic tests.

HIV-2 and the simian immunodeficiency viruses (SIVs) form a subgroup of more closely related viruses (greater than 80% sequence identity) that are divergent from the HIV-1s. An SIV isolated from mandrills (SIV_{MND}) appears to be equally related to HIV-1 and HIV-2.[10] Another HIV-like virus recently isolated from a chimpanzee caught in the wild exhibits sequence identity more closely related to HIV-1 than to HIV-2.[11]

TABLE 3.2 HIV characteristics that resemble those of lentiviruses.

Biology
Persistent or latent infection
Cytopathic effects (syncitia formation) on selected cells
Capable of infecting macrophages
Associated with immune suppression
Long incubation period
Central nervous system involvement
Affects hematopoietic system
Molecular Biology
Similar genomic organization
Morphology of virus (cylindrical nucleoid)
Accumulation of unintegrated proviral DNA
Polymorphism, particularly in the envelope gene
Primer binding site ($tRNA^{lys}$)

Structure of HIV

The structure of HIV resembles that of all retroviruses but particularly that of the lentiviruses (Figure 3.2). HIV has a cylindrical, eccentric nucleoid or core. The nucleoid contains the HIV genome, which is diploid, that is, composed of two identical single-stranded RNAs. Encoded in the RNA genome are the entire complement of genes of the virus. These genes code for (contain the genetic information for) the structural proteins, which are used to assemble the virus particles, and the regulatory proteins involved in the regulation of viral gene expression (Table 3.3 and Figure 3.3).

The HIV RNA genome is associated with a basic nucleic acid-binding protein p9 and the reverse (RT) (see Figure 3.2). The core or capsid antigen p24 encloses the nucleoid components, completing the nucleocapsid structure. The matrix antigen p17 encircles the viral core and lines

TABLE 3.3. Summary of HIV proteins.

Gene product	Description
env (envelope)	
gp160	Precursor of *env* glycoprotein
gp120	Outer *env* glycoprotein
gp41	Transmembrane glycoprotein
gag (core)	
p55	Precursor of *gag* proteins
p24	*gag* protein
p17	*gag* protein
p15, p9, p7	*gag* protein
pol (polymerase)	
p66	Reverse transcriptase of *pol* gene
p51	Reverse transcriptase of *pol* gene
p31	Endonuclease of *pol* gene
tat (transactivator)	Transactivator of viral proteins (formerly *tat*-3)
p14	
rev (regulator)	Regulates expression of virus proteins (formerly *art* or *trs*)
p19/20	
vif (infectivity factor)	Determines virus infectivity (formerly *sor*)
p23	
vpr (R)	Unknown (formerly R)
nef (negative factor)	Reduces virus expression
p27	
vpu (only in HIV-1)	Reduces amount of virus released from cells
p16	
vpx (only in HIV-2)	Unknown
p14	

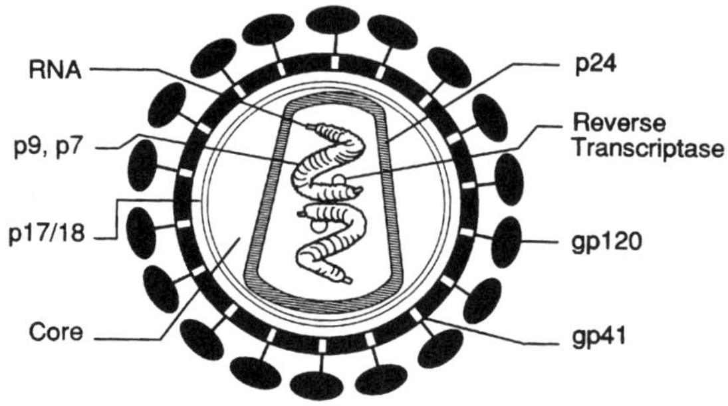

FIGURE 3.2. Schematic representation of morphologic structure of HIV-1 in cross section.

the inner surface of the envelope of the virus. The surface of HIV manifests external knoblike structures formed by the envelope glycoprotein (sugar-containing protein) gp120. The transmembrane protein (TMP) gp41 spans the viral membrane and has both external and internal domains. The TMP anchors the external gp120 to the viral envelope. The membrane lipid bilayer is derived from the host cell plasma membrane.

The envelope gene (*env*) of HIV codes for a precursor polyprotein p85, which is glycosylated to form the *env* precursor protein gp160 (Figure 3.4). The gp160 is then cleaved by a cellular protease to form the surface

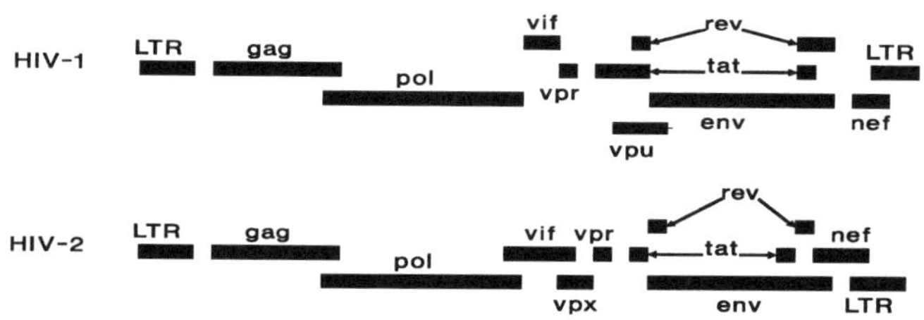

GENE	FUNCTION
GAG	CORE PROTEINS
POL	ENZYMES (RT, PROTEASE, INTEGRASE)
ENV	ENVELOPE PROTEINS
TAT	POSITIVE REGULATOR
REV	DIFFERENTIAL REGULATOR
VIF	INFECTIVITY FACTOR
VPR	NOT KNOWN
VPU (HIV-1 ONLY)	NOT KNOWN
VPX (HIV-2 ONLY)	NOT KNOWN
NEF	NEGATIVE REGULATOR?

FIGURE 3.3. Structure of genomes of HIV-1 and HIV-2 with individual viral genes and functions.

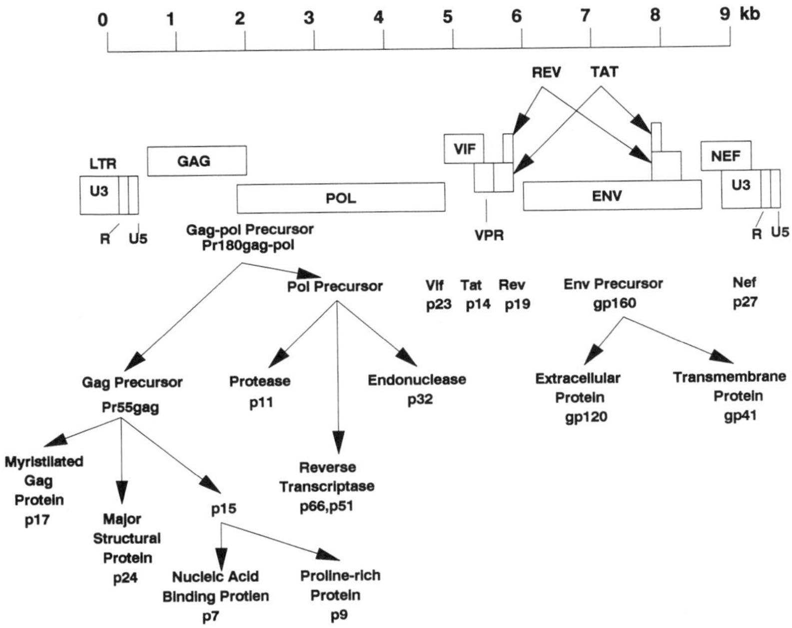

FIGURE 3.4. Schematic of synthesis and processing of proteins coded for by HIV-1 genome.

virion extracellular envelope glycoprotein gp120 and the TMP gp41.[12] The gp120 protein contains specific amino acid domains responsible for binding the virus to the CD4 virus receptor protein on the surface of the cell. The gp41 protein contains stretches of amino acids that play an important role in syncytia formation. Fusion, mediated by the gp41 TMP, may also play a role in the penetration of the viral core into the interior of the cell. Another domain of the TMP spans the membrane and anchors the envelope gp120 protein onto the infected cell or virus particle.

The *gag* gene encodes a 55-kd (kilodalton) polyprotein precursor molecule (Pr55*gag*) that is cleaved into the major structural proteins of the virus capsid (p17 and p25) and core structures (p15, which is further cleaved to p7 and p9) surrounding the virion RNA. During the synthesis of the Pr55*gag* polyprotein, the fatty acid myristate is attached to the amino terminal end (p17) of the precursor protein. Myristoylation of Pr55*gag* appears to be required for production of infectious virions.[13] The p9 protein contains multiple cysteine residues that probably help to form the specific secondary necessary for nucleic acid binding. The function of the proline-rich virion core protein p9 remains unclear.

A second polyprotein precursor, the Pr180*gag-pol*, contains the *gag*, protease, polymerase, and integrase gene products translated from the same genomic messenger RNA as the *gag* polyprotein Pr55*gag*. The pol part of the message actually codes for three proteins that are cleaved from the larger precursor molecule (Pr180*gag-pol*). These include the protease, the reverse transcriptase (RT), and integrase. The viral protease is involved in the processing of the Pr180*gag-pol* and the Pr55*gag*.[14] Cleavage of the *gag-pol* precursor by a functional protease releases the RT and integrase.

Life Cycle of HIV

The first step in the infection of a susceptible cell is the attachment of HIV to the cell through a specific interaction of the viral envelope glycoprotein gp120 with the cell-surface-associated CD4 protein (Figure 3.5). The TMP gp41 noncovalently interacts with the gp120 and is involved in virus–cell and cell–cell fusion events. Jointly these two HIV surface proteins are responsible for virion binding of CD4-bearing cells and for syncytia formation between infected and uninfected cells. The binding step to the CD4 receptor protein could potentially be inhibited by anti-gp120 virus-neutralizing antibodies (Figure 3.5). After binding of the virus to the CD4 protein of the cell, penetration of the virus capsid into the cell occurs by fusion of the viral and cellular membranes. Infection seems to be species specific, because murine cells with the human CD4 antigen bind but do not take up HIV.

After the virus is internalized it is partially uncoated, thereby activating the viral RT that converts the single-stranded viral RNA into double-

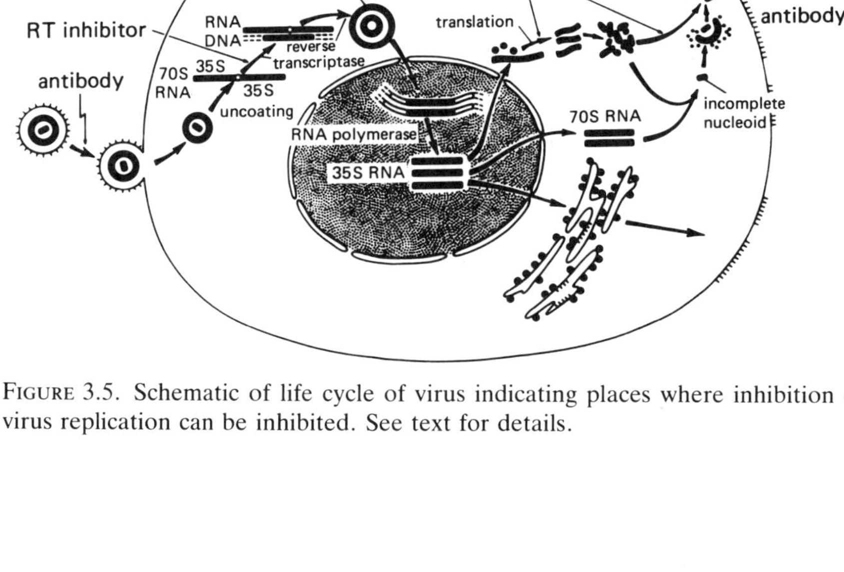

FIGURE 3.5. Schematic of life cycle of virus indicating places where inhibition of virus replication can be inhibited. See text for details.

stranded linear DNA. This step can be inhibited by compounds such as azidothymidime (zidovudine), which are RT inhibitors that prematurely terminate the growing DNA chain preventing formation of the HIV provirus (see Figure 3.5). The DNA product is then transported from the cytoplasm of the cell to the nucleus. It is believed that the linear, rather than a circular form, becomes the integrated provirus.[15] The integration of the linear viral DNA into the host's chromosomes is mediated by the virus-coded integrase.

HIV gene expression involves synthesis of viral messenger RNA (mRNA) transcripts using the host cell's RNA polymerase II and other cellular and viral transcriptional factors. The mRNAs for the *gag* and *gag-pol* precursors and for the viral RNA present in the mature virions represent full-length transcripts of the viral genome. A smaller, singly spliced transcript codes for the envelope components. The regulatory proteins of HIV (nef, rev, tat, vif, vpr) are synthesized via translation from multiply spliced transcripts that are not found in the viral particle. However, they do play a significant role in virus expression.[16] The control of HIV replication is regulated through the interplay of the regulatory gene products, and specific sequences present in the viral RNA or provirus.[17] The proportion of the different mRNAs transported from the nucleus to the cytoplasm for translation into viral proteins is determined by the regulatory protein encoded by the HIV *rev* gene.

Assembly of the newly synthesized virion occurs in the cytoplasm and involves formation of a dimer of identical viral RNA molecules in a complex containing *gag* and *pol* gene products. The synthesis and assembly of the virion components could be potentially inhibited by compounds such as interferon (see Figure 3.5). The resulting core structure buds from the cellular membrane where it acquires its envelope glycoprotein coat (consisting of gp120 and gp41) and a cellular lipid bilayer. Cleavage of the internal core proteins by the viral protease occurs during this process, yielding extracellular infectious progeny HIVs. The extracellular virus could potentially be attacked and destroyed at this stage by sensitized T-cell antibodies (see Figure 3.5). Infectious HIV can undergo cell-to-cell spread, independent of virus release, through the fusion or syncytia formation of an infected cell with an uninfected cell.

The mechanism for HIV latency is still unclear. However, it is known that the level of HIV replication is strikingly affected by activation of resting lymphocytes. Resting T cells are nonpermissive for the replication of HIV-1 despite efficient binding of the virus to the CD4 receptor molecule displayed at the surface of the cell. The transition from a latent to a productive infection has been suggested to occur in response to T-cell mitogens, phorbol esters, calcium ionophores, and gene products of other viruses such as HTLV-I, herpes simplex viruses, cytomegalovirus, adenovirus, hepatitis B virus, and human herpesvirus-6. T-cell activation is important for virus penetration. Once the host cell is activated, inducible

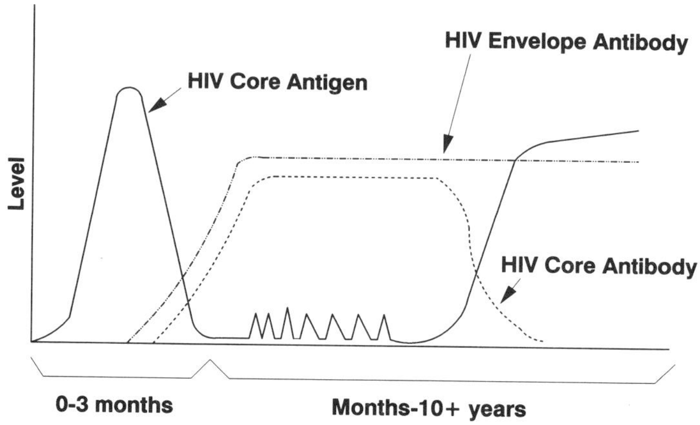

FIGURE 3.6. Temporal serologic relationship between HIV-1 antigen (p24) production and detection of HIV-specific antibodies.

host cell transcription (the process of conversion of DNA to RNA) factors stimulate a low level of early HIV-1 gene expression. The first mRNA molecules that reach the cytoplasm from the nucleus are composed entirely of multiply spliced messages that code for the HIV-1 regulatory proteins. Once the *tat* protein is produced it elicits a strong positive effect on viral transcription. *Tat* acts by increasing the rate of transcription of all the gene sequences linked to the HIV LTR (long terminal repeat).

In Vivo HIV Infectivity

HIV infection of susceptible cells in a person occurs via interaction of the external membrane glycoprotein gp120 on the virus and the cell-surface receptor, CD4. The primary CD4-bearing cells in HIV-infected persons are the T-helper lymphocytes, selected marrow progenitor cells, and monocytes and macrophages. Additionally, a variety of nonhematopoietic cells expressing low levels of CD4 on their surface are also susceptible to HIV infection.[18] These include the epidermal Langerhans cells, follicular dentritic cells of lymph nodes, and certain cells of the central nervous system. Interestingly, infection of glial cell lines, colorectal cells, and fetal brain cells, which do not appear to express detectable surface CD4, suggests that another mechanism may also be responsible for virus infection.[19]

During the first several weeks following infection with HIV, a brief period of acute viremia and p24 antigenemia occurs and can be detected in the plasma of infected persons (Figure 3.6).

During this period, patients also may experience an acute mononucleosis-like illness. In most infections, the antigen becomes undetectable when antibodies to p24 emerge, although antigen may appear later in the course before the development of AIDS. Transient IgM and persistent IgG and IgA antibodies to a broad range of virus-encoded proteins can be detected. Although there have been reports of delayed antibody response to HIV-1 infection, 95% or more of infected persons develop detectable antibodies to HIV-1 within 3 to 6 months.[20] The interval between infection and seroconversion or detection of antibodies has been called the "window period." This period has received much attention because of implications for the safety of the blood supply and the possibility of allowing HIV-1-infected seronegative blood to be used for transfusion. Recent studies of more than 1 million blood donors in the United States, West Germany, and Austria have failed to demonstrate a single instance of an antigen-positive, antibody-negative collection, presumable because antigenemia is short lived in relation to the time between infection and donation. This result implies that routine use of a screening test for HIV antigen would not increase the safety of the blood supply.

The acute phase of HIV infection is commonly followed by a long period (up to 10 years or more) of low-level viremia and chronic subacute infection. Disease symptoms are usually mild or unapparent during this period. Viral antigen or cell-free virus can only be intermittently detected in the circulation, and high titers of antibodies to the viral *env*, *gag*, and *pol* proteins are usually present in the patient's serum or plasma, saliva, and cerebrospinal fluid (CSF). The last phase of infection is characterized by increased virus expression and spread, and the onset of multiple disease symptoms indicative of AIDS. By this time, the patients have a severely depleted level of CD4-positive T-helper cells leading to collapse of their immune system. There is also a decrease in HIV-specific antibodies (usually anti-p24 *gag* antibodies) and an increase in p24 antigenemia. Even though virus-neutralizing antibodies can be identified in sera from certain patients at all stages of infection, this does not correlate well with their clinical status.

Although HIV has been isolated from saliva, tears, and urine, the presence of infected cells or cell-free virus is rare, and there is no evidence that exposure to these body fluids represents a significant risk of infection. In contrast, virus has been isolated more frequently from the peripheral blood mononuclear cells of patients. In general, the percentage of patients producing antibody to HIV-1 who will also have positive peripheral blood cultures varies as a function of both the severity of infection and the methods employed to optimize the detection of positive cultures. Recently, it has been shown that with optimization of technique at all levels more than 90–95% of HIV-1-infected persons may have positive cocultures regardless of CD4 count or clinical staging.[21]

Conclusion

It has been a reltively short time since the initial identification of HIV. In that time, extraordinary progress has been made in our understanding of the viral and cellular mechanisms governing infection and replication. However, major gaps in our knowledge of HIV infection, latency, replication, and pathogenesis persist, and many essential questions remain to be answered. These include: (i) the nature of the latent state of infection that is believed to exist in vivo; (ii) the nature of viral and host factors involved in viral latency; (iii) the nature of the molecular events involved in virus-induced cell killing; and (iv) the nature of the genetic differences for different HIV variants involved in differential virus replication, tissue tropism, and cytopathogenicity. The answers to these and other critical questions are vital to our understanding of the HIV disease process and to the development of effective new treatments and vaccine strategies against this devastating viral disease.

References

1. Barre-Sinoussi F, Chermann JC, Rey F, Nugeyre MT, Chamaret S, Gruest J, Dauguet C, Axler-Blin C, Brun-Vezinet F, Rouzioux C, Rozenbaum W, Montagnier L. Isolation of a T-lymphotropic retrovirus from a patient at risk for acquired immune deficiency syndrome (AIDS). Science 1983;220: 868–871.
2. Gallo RC, Salahuddin SZ, Popovic M, Shearer GM, Kaplan M, Hayres BF, Palker TJ, Redfield R, Oleske J, Safai B, White G, Foster P, Markham P. Frequent detection and isolation of cytopathic retroviruses (HTLV-III) from patients with AIDS and at-risk for AIDS. Science 1984;224:500–502.
3. Popovic M, Sarngadharan MG, Read E, Gallo RC. Detection, isolation and continuous production of cytopathic retroviruses (HTLV-III) from patients with AIDS and pre-AIDS. Science 1984;224:297–500.
4. Clavel F. HIV-2, the West African AIDS virus. AIDS 1987;1:135–140.
5. Clavel F, Guetard D, Brun-Vezinet F, Chamaret S, Rey M, Santos-Ferreira MO, Laurent AG, Dauget C, Katlama C, Rouzioux C Klatzmann, D Champalimaud JL, Montagnier L. Isolation of a new human retrovirus from West African patients with AIDS. Science 1986;233:343–346.
6. Horsburgh CR, Holmberg SD. The global distribution human immunodeficiency virus type 2 (HIV-2) infection. Transfusion (Philadelphia) 1988;28: 192–195.
7. Varmus H. Retroviruses. Science 1988;240:1427–1435.
8. Alizon M, Wain-Hobson S, Montagnier L, Sonigo P. Genetic variability of the AIDS virus: nucleotide sequence analysis of two isolates from African patients. Cell 1986;46:63–74.
9. Clavel F, Guyader M, Guetard D, Salle M, Montagnier L, Alizon M. Molecular cloning and polymorphism of the human immunodeficiency virus type 2. Nature (London) 1986;324:691–695.

10. Tsujimoto H, Hasegawa H, Maki N, Fukasawa M, Miura T, Speidel S, Cooper RW, Moriyama LN, Gojoburi T, Hayami, M. Sequence of a novel simian immunodeficiency virus from a wild-caught African mandrill. Nature (London) 1989;341:539–541.
11. Peeters M, Honore C, Huet T, Bedjabaga L, Ossati S, Bussi P, Cooper RW, Delaporte E. Isolation and partial characterization of an HIV-related virus occurring naturally in chimpanzees in Gabon. AIDS 1989;3:625–630.
12. Haseltine WA. Development of antiviral drugs for the treatment of AIDS: strategies and prospects. J Acquired Immune Deficiency Syndromes 1989;2: 311–334.
13. Bryant ML, Ratner L. Myristoylation-dependent replication and assembly of human immunodeficiency virus 1. Proc Natl Acad Sci USA 1990;87:523–527.
14. Debouck C, Gorniak JG, Stickler JE, Metcalf BW, Rosenberg M. Human immunodeficiency virus protease expresses in *Escherichia coli* exhibits autoprocessing and specific maturation of the gag precursor. Proc Natl Acad Sci USA 1987;84:8903–8906.
15. Fujiwara T, Mizuuchi K. Retroviral DNA integration: structure of an integration intermediate. Cell 1988;54:497–504.
16. Peerlin BM, Luciw PA. Molecular biology of HIV. AIDS 1988;2(Suppl 1):S29–S40.
17. Cullen BR, Greene WC. Regulatory pathways governing HIV-1 replication. Cell 1989;58:423–426.
18. Levy JA. 1989. Human immunodeficiency viruses and the pathogenesis of AIDS. JAMA 1989;261:2997–3006.
19. Takeda A, Tuazon CU, Ennis FA. Antibody-enhanced infection by HIV-1 via Fc receptor-mediated entry. Science 1988;242:580–583.
20. Horsburgh CR Jr., Ou C-Y, Jason J, et al. Duration of human immunodeficiency virus infection before detection of antibody. Lancet 1989;2:637–640.
21. Coombs RW, Collier AC, Allain J-P, Nikora, B, Leuther H, Gjerset GF, Corey L. Plasma viremia in human immunodeficiency virus infection. N Engl J Med 1989;321:1626–1631.

4
Immunologic Aspects of Human Immunodeficiency Virus Infection

ALISON C. MAWLE and J. STEVEN McDOUGAL

The human immunodeficiency virus (HIV-1) infects, functionally impairs, and depletes a subpopulation of thymus-derived T lymphocytes that express that cell-surface molecule CD4. CD4 T cells perform critical recognition and induction functions in the immune response to foreign stimuli. Infection results in gradual CD4 T-cell depletion, progressive immune unresponsiveness with effective paralysis in virtually all arms of the immune system, and increasing susceptibility to opportunistic infections and malignancies. The clinical spectrum of HIV infection ranges from asymptomatic infection to severe immunodeficiency with the infectious/malignant complications that are characteristic of the acquired immunodeficiency syndrome (AIDS). This spectrum of clinical severity is reflected in a parallel severity of CD4 T-cell depletion. HIV-infected people mount and sustain a vigorous immune response to HIV. However, it remains unclear what role the immune response has in controlling HIV infection, and, more importantly, which components of the immune response effectively combat infection/progression. The study of the immune response in this setting is difficult because the cells involved in initiating an immune response are the same cells that are infected by HIV.

In summary, HIV-1 immunodeficiency is viewed from the immunologic perspective as a graded severity of CD4 T-cell depletion, distributed on a continuum of time, influenced by incompletely understood cofactors, and associated with a spectrum of increasing clinical severity that reflects the severity of CD4 T-cell depletion. Unlike the immunodeficiency syndrome, the other major clinical sequela of HIV infection, subacute encephalopathy, is not necessarily related to the degree of CD4 T-cell depletion. However, as we shall see, a common immunopathologic mechanism is involved: infection of a monocyte-derived cell type that expresses the CD4 molecule.

Organization of the Immune System

The function of the immune system is to discriminate self from nonself. As a consequence of nonself recognition, cellular and humoral interactions are set in motion that result in the sequestration and elimination of that which is recognized as foreign or antigenic. The immune response has the features of specificity (ability to discriminate related antigens), memory (a more rapid and heightened response on secondary exposure to antigen), recruitment (induction of secondary antigen-nonspecific mechanisms of antigen disposal), and regulation (dampening or amplification).

The immune system is derived from two cell lineages: monocytic and lymphocytic. Monocytes and their tissue counterparts, macrophages, seed structures of the mononuclear phagocytic system (Kupffer's cells, sinusoidal cells in the spleen, Langerhan's cells in the skin, microglial cells in the brain, dendritic cells in lymph nodes and thymus, etc.). These cells have no innate antigen specificity but do scavenge antigens (especially particulate antigens) and present them in an immunogenic form to lymphoid cells. By virtue of receptors for immunoglobulin, complement, or lymphokines, they respond to mediators of the immune response and are recruited to mount an inflammatory attack on foreign antigens.

Lymphocytes are divided into two major types (Table 4.1): T cells and B cells. B cells are derived from bone marrow (and fetal liver). They synthesize immunoglobulin and express it on their cell surface as integral membrane immunoglobulin (sIg). Although sIg defines B cells, another surface structure, CD20, detected with monoclonal antibodies, is often used for enumerating this population. B cells are not actively engaged in the secretion of immunoglobulins. Rather, they are precursor cells that, after appropriate antigen recognition and stimulation, proliferate and differentiate to become memory B cells or plasma cells. The latter are actively engaged in secretion of Ig and are the source of serum immunoglobulins. B cells comprise about 10% of peripheral blood lymphocytes. However, they compose 50% of cells that populate lymphoid organs such as the lymph nodes, where they are organized in follicles.

T cells are also bone-marrow-derived cells. They require the presence of an intact thymus for development of immunocompetence. After migration to the thymus, they undergo a series of differentiation and selection steps. Here, self-reactive cells are either eliminated or paralyzed (negative selection or tolerance induction) or the cells acquire immunocompetence and emerge with cell-surface markers characteristic of mature peripheral blood T cells (positive selection). The selection process is highly abortive: only 10% of precursor cells that populate the thymus emerge as peripheral T cells.

Mature T cells represent nearly 90% of peripheral blood lymphocytes. These cells circulate from blood to tissue to lymph. They are relatively

TABLE 4.1 Lymphocyte cell-surface markers.

Cell type	Marker	Function
T cell	CD 3	T-cell–receptor complex
	CD2	Cell–cell adhesion; sheep red blood cell receptor
	CD4	T-helper cell; interacts with MHC class II
	CD8	T-cytotoxic and T-suppressor cells; interact with MHC class I
	CD4/CD8	Immature T cell; predominantly in thymus
T-cell subsets	CD4 CD45RA	Naive T-helper cells
	CD4 CD29	Memory T-helper cells
	CD8 $CD11b^-$	Cytotoxic T cells
	CD8 $CD11b^+$	Suppressor T cells
Activated T cell	CD25	IL2 receptor
	CD38	T-cell activation marker
	MHC class II (Ia)	
B cell	MHC class II (Ia)	Presents antigen to CD4 cells
	sIg	Surface immunoglobulin; binds antigen
	CD20	B-cell accessory molecule
Natural killer (NK) cell	CD56	Unknown
	CD16	Fc receptor
All lymphocytes	MHC class I	Presents antigen to CD8 cells

long lived, and their recirculation pattern is ideally suited for immune surveillance. Mature T cells posses a variety of cell-surface structures that can be detected with monoclonal antibodies. Two T-cell markers, CD2 and CD3, are found on most mature T cells and are referred to as pan-T-cell markers. CD2 is involved in intercellular adhesion and antigen-independent activation of T cells. CD3 is a polypeptide structure that is physically associated with the T-cell receptor (TCR) for antigen. It mediates intracellular signal transduction and activation following antigen recognition by the TCR.

CD2/CD3 T cells can be further subdivided by two other phenotypic markers, CD4 and CD8. During T-cell ontogeny in the thymus, double CD4/CD8-positive cells exist, which lose one or the other marker to become mature T cells. These markers are on mutually exclusive T-cell populations in the periphery. (Rare double-positive cells can sometimes be found in the periphery.) Historically, CD4 and CD8 T-cell populations have been associated with helper/inducer and cytotoxic/suppressor functions, respectively. This remains a predominant association, although it is by no means absolute. A more stringent association of CD4 or CD8 phenotype with function is in the mode by which they recognize antigen rather than in their subsequent effector functions. CD4 T cells recognize antigen that is processed and presented in the context of class II structures of the major histocompatibility complex (MHC), that is, HLA-DR, HLA-DP, or HLA-DQ. CD8 T cells recognize antigen in the context of class I MHC structures, that is, HLA-A, HLA-B, or HLA-C.

When antigen is introduced into a host, a humoral (antibody) response or a cellular immune response or both may ensue, and both these involve cell–cell interactions between multiple cell types. The B-cell (antibody) response is a case in point. Although the specificity of the surface immunoglobulin on a given B cell is identical to the specificity of the antibody secreted by its progeny, the plasma cell, simple interaction of antigen with B cells is not sufficient to induce antibody formation. For all but a few so-called T-independent antigens, there is a requirement for T-cell recognition of processed antigen and T-cell stimulation of the B-cell response.

Antigen recognition by B cells and T cells is fundamentally different. B-cell surface immunoglobulin or serum antibody binds directly to native antigen. In contrast, T cells generally do not recognize native antigen; rather, they recognize antigen that is processed and presented in association with MHC class I or II molecules by antigen-presenting cells (APC). Antigen processing is poorly understood. There is a preferential presentation of endogenously produced antigens (i.e., antigens produced by intracellular pathogens such as viruses) with class I MHC. Exogenously introduced antigens tend to be presented in the context of class II MHC. This distinction is by no means rigid. T cells recognize both processed antigen and MHC, that is, their response to antigen is restricted by the MHC (MHC restriction). Antigen–MHC recognition is performed by the TCR, which recognizes antigen bound in a pocket of the MHC molecule. Most nucleated cells express class I molecules and can present antigen to or be recognized by CD8 T cells. MHC class II has a more limited cellular distribution, being confined to cells of monocyte lineage and B cells. The latter are very potent APC for CD4 T cells (a particularly potent combination is B cells and CD4 T cells specific for different epitopes on the same antigen). Some cell types that normally do not express MHC class II do so when activated (T cells) or stimulated by an inflammatory response (epithelial cells). After antigen recognition by the T cell, signals are transmitted to the interior via CD3, and this sets in motion the biochemical events required for the effector phase of the particular T cell's function.

CD4 and CD8 T cells exist in peripheral blood in a ratio of 2:1 (range 1:1 to 3:1). CD4 T cells are a pivotal cell in the orchestration of an effective immune response. They mount the initial specific response to processed antigen (presented in the context of class II MHC) and, in turn, induce other cells to perform their respective immunologic functions. They do this through cell–cell contact or the elaboration of mediators (lymphokines). They induce cytotoxic CD8 T cells, which recognize antigens presented on class I MHC and lyse the presenting cell. Through the elaboration of lymphokines, CD4 T cells can recruit inflammatory cells, particularly macrophages (delayed-type hypersensitivity response). They induce antigen-specific B cells to proliferate and differentiate into plasma cells secreting specific antibody. Finally, they induce CD8 suppressor cells that regulate the amplitude of the immune response at multiple levels.

CD4 and CD8 T cells have been further subdivided using monoclonal antibodies directed at other cell-surface markers: CD45R (2H4) or CD29 (4B4) identify helper cells that induce CD8 cells or B cells. CD11b (Leu15) is used to distinguish CD8 suppressor cells ($CD11b^+$) from cytotoxic cells ($CD11b^-$). At this time, these subpopulations markers do not have particularly relevant clinical or diagnostic usefulness. After antigen-specific or nonspecific (mitogenic) stimulation, T cells of either the CD8 or CD4 T-cell subclass express new markers not present on resting T cells. Among these are class II MHC structures (HLA-DR) and a receptor for the T-cell growth factor interleukin 2 (IL-2). These markers have been used to assess the degree of T-cell stimulation.

A numerically minor proportion of lymphocytes do not fit any of the three phenotypic categories already discussed, namely sIg-positive B cells and the CD4 or CD8 subsets of CD2/CD3 T cells. These are commonly (and inappropriately) referred to as null cells. Most null cells have receptors for complement or for immunoglobulin, and most null cells are natural killer (NK) cells. NK cells are large granular lymphocytes (LGL) that can kill a variety of tumor cell lines in vitro. This activity is nonspecific in the sense that it does not require prior sensitization nor is it MHC restricted. These features distinguish NK cells from CD8 cytolytic T cells. It is also distinguished from the activity of another group of "null" cells, K cells, that mediate antibody-dependent cellular cytotoxicity (ADCC). K cells have receptors for immunoglobulin (FcR). They recognize and lyse antibody-coated target cells. NK and K cells defy easy phenotypic classification. The majority of NK cells express the NKH1 (CD56) markers, are CD3/CD4/CD8 negative, and do not use antibody or the conventional TCR for cellular recognition. A minority may express low levels of CD3, CD8, and a TCR, and are distinguished functionally from cytolytic CD8 cells in that they are MHC unrestricted in their activity.

Cellular Tropism of HIV-1

All mammalian cells that have been tested have an inherent capacity to replicate infectious HIV provided HIV is introduced as cloned and integrated proviral DNA by transfection.[1-3] Therefore, the apparent preferential tropism of HIV for certain cell types must relate to events that occur before replication (attachment, penetration, reverse transcription, or integration). Infection by exogenous HIV has been most reliably and reproducibly demonstrated in cells that express CD4. Preferential infectivity for CD4-positive cells has been demonstrated using separated normal human cell populations as well as continuous cell lines,[4–6] and virus is most readily isolated or detected in CD4 cells from HIV-infected people although infectivity for some CD4-negative cell lines has been reported.[7]

The CD4 molecule has binding avidity for the gp120 outer envelope protein of HIV-1, and this appears to be the major determinant of cellular susceptibility to natural infection by HIV-1. Evidence that CD4 functions as a receptor for HIV-1 comes from several lines of investigation. Monoclonal antibodies to CD4 prevent infection of CD4 cells by HIV-1.[6,8,9] Virus binds specifically to CD4 cells, and this binding is inhibited by anti-CD4 or anti-gp120 antibodies.[10] Bimolecular complexes of CD4 and gp120 are isolated from HIV-1-exposed CD4 T cells.[11] Human cells that do not express CD4 and cannot be infected by HIV-1 are rendered susceptible by transfection and expression of CD4 cDNA.[12] Finally, soluble forms of the CD4 molecule block HIV binding and infectivity.[13]

All cells expressing the CD4 molecule have been shown to be infectable with the virus in vitro. In addition to T cells and T-cell lines, this includes monocytes that may serve as a reservoir of infection in the body,[14,15] monocyte cell lines[16] Epstein–Barr virus- (EBV-) transformed B-cell lines,[17] and glial cell lines.[18] Infectivity for some CD4-negative cell lines has also been reported.

Mechanisms of CD4 T-Cell Depletion

The precise mechanism by which HIV-1 infection causes CD4 cell death remains obscure. Reasonable hypotheses derived from other viral systems include the following. Massive budding of virus from the membrane results in cell lysis. Massive viral replication commandeers cellular transcriptional/translational machinery required for maintenance of cellular integrity. Viral infection somehow initiates normal cellular processes that result in terminal differentiation and senescence, the so-called programmed cell death that is associated with DNA fragmentation (apoptosis). Both in vitro studies and clinical studies support the notion that increased viral replication is associated with more rapid CD4 T-cell depletion, which in turn may be determined by the activation state of the infected cells. However, any model of cell death must take into account an additional unique feature of this virus, its interaction with CD4.

The basic observation, based on genetic manipulation of virus and its introduction into various cell types, is that the minimum and sufficient requirements for cytopathicity is *env* gene expression by the virus *and* CD4 expression by the infected cell. Introduction of HIV-1 into CD4-negative cells by transfection results in equivalent viral replication but no cell death.[19] Similarly, certain *env* mutants that cannot bind CD4 will replicate if introduced into CD4 cells, but cell death does not ensue.[20] Intracellular complexes of envelope and CD4 proteins accumulate in HIV-1-infected cells, interfering with transport of CD4 to the cell surface, and these may somehow be toxic to the cell.[7]

Mechanisms of CD4 T-cell depletion that do not require productive infection by the doomed CD4 T cell have also been proposed. Infected cells fuse and form syncytia with uninfected CD4 cells, a phenomenon presumed tantamount to cell death. *Env* gene expression is required of the infected cell, and CD4 expression is required of its fusion partner.[21,22] It has been argued that a mechanism by which infected cells sequester uninfected cells may explain how massive CD4 T-cell depletion can occur when so few cells with demonstrable HIV-1 are detected in vivo. However, the relative importance of syncytia formation versus direct viral destruction of individually infected cells in explaining CD4 T-cell depletion remains to be determined.

The outer envelope protein gp120 is readily shed in soluble form from virions and infected cells, and it retains CD4 binding activity. Several mechanisms by which soluble gp120 impairs CD4 T-cell function or mediates CD4 T-cell destruction have been proposed. CD4 cells coated with gp120 react with anti-gp120 antibodies and serve as targets for antibody-dependent cellular cytotoxicity (ADCC).[23] Cells armed with anti-gp120 antibodies that mediate ADCC are frequently found in HIV-1-infected people.[24] By virtue of binding and internalization, CD4 T cells can process and present gp120 peptides for recognition by gp120-specific, MHC-restricted cytolytic T cells.[25] Finally, gp120 bound to CD4 may theoretically interfere with normal functions of CD4 such as MHC class II recognition. Immunosuppressive effects of gp120 on CD4 T-cell function have been described in vitro.[26]

Autoimmune phenomena may occur in the course of HIV infection and have been offered as possible mechanisms of T-cell destruction. Autoantibodies to T cells have been demonstrated. Similarly, the possibility that the antibody response to the binding site of gp120 sets up an idiotypic-antiidiotypic cascade that ultimately results in anti-CD4 reactive antibodies has theoretical appeal but no practical demonstration. Antibodies that react with soluble forms of CD4 can be detected in about 10% of HIV-1-infected people. They bear no relation to disease progression; they do not react with the site on CD4 involved in binding gp120, nor do they react with CD4 in its native conformation on the cell surface.[27]

Major Components of the Immune System in HIV-1 Infection

CD4 T Cells and CD4/CD8 Ratio

A low ratio of CD4 to CD8 T cells has been a characteristic and consistent observation since the earliest reports of AIDS. Inverted ratios result from a decrease in the absolute number of CD4 T cells and a variable number (increase, normal, or decrease) of CD8 T cells.[28] The infectivity of HIV-1 for CD4 T cells predicts that numerical depletion of CD4 T cells would reflect the primary lesion more accurately than CD4/CD8 ratio. However, both have their place in the evaluation of HIV-1-infected people.

In early infection and in asymptomatic infection, ratio is more sensitive to reciprocal changes in CD4 and CD8 cell counts that occur, whereas abnormally low CD4 cell counts are unusual. For example, an infectious mononucleosis-like syndrome has been described in association with acute HIV-1 infection and seroconversion. CD4/CD8 ratios are generally low (because CD8 counts are elevated) whereas CD4 cell counts tend to be normal or low normal.[29] In studies comparing uninfected and infected risk group members who are asymptomatic, CD4/CD8 ratio is a much more sensitive indicator of HIV-1 infection than absolute CD4 T-cell count. Subjects with common but less severe clinical manifestations have abnormalities intermediate between those of AIDS patients and seropositive, asymptomatic risk group members.

Although CD4/CD8 ratio is a more sensitive indicator of HIV-1 infection, absolute CD4 T-cell count is a more specific marker for severe immunodeficiency with clinical complications.[30,31] Abnormally low CD4 T-cell counts are found in most AIDS patients at diagnosis (65–95%), and virtually all patients who survive long enough will eventually develop this abnormality. Low CD4 cell counts are unusual in asymptomatic, infected people (<5%) and infrequent in AIDS-related complex (ARC) (<20%). When a low level of CD4 T cells occurs in these settings, it is a poor prognostic sign. Patients with Kaposi's sarcoma as the sole manifestation of disease tend to have less severe abnormalities than those with opportunistic infections. Those who recover from opportunistic infections generally have more CD4 T cells than those who do not, and once the diagnosis of AIDS is made, progressive depletion of CD4 T cells with time is the rule.

Clinically, a reasonable case can be made for the use of CD4 T-cell determinations for monitoring HIV-1-infected patients, because these cells are the primary target of infection and their depletion reflects the severity of immunosuppression better than any other test. CD4 cell counts have been used for stratifying patients for entrance into clinical trials.

They will most certainly also be used for assessing the response to therapy. In therapeutic trials, clinical outcome is the generally accepted measurement of therapeutic response; however, measurement of CD4 cell levels is an objective additional measure that has been promoted as a rational surrogate.

CD4 T cells are functionally and phenotypically heterogeneous. Preferential loss of certain subsets in vivo has been reported.[28,32] Moreover, surviving CD4 T cells, on a per cell basis, may show selective defects in some in vitro assays such as antigen-induced proliferation or the autologous mixed lymphocyte reaction, whereas responses to pan-T-cell mitogens are intact.[33] Antigen-specific proliferation is believed to be an in vitro correlate of delayed-type hypersensitivity, and skin test responses tend to be impaired in HIV-1-infected patients, especially in advanced disease.

The reason for CD4 phenotypic or functional imbalances early in infection is obscure. There is some evidence for preferential infectivity HIV-1 of the $CD29^+$ CD4 memory subset both in vivo and in vitro, which may account for loss of antigen-specific responses.[34] Some of the functional defects can be reproduced in normal cells with HIV-1 gp120.[26] In any event, these phenotypic/functional imbalances do not appear to have strong prognostic significance. More appropriately stated, they do not outperform enumeration of total CD4 T cells in reflecting clinical status.

CD8 T Cells

CD8 T cells may be normal, elevated, or depressed in number. Elevations are more frequent early in infection and in asymptomatic subjects, whereas in endstage disease CD8 T cells may decline in parallel with CD4 T cells, resulting in panlymphopenia. There is no evidence that normal CD8 cells are susceptible to natural infection with HIV-1. Although HIV-1 introduced into CD8 cells will replicate, it is not cytopathic.[19] CD8 T cells depend on CD4 T cells for induction of effector functions and possibly for maintenance of precursor numbers as well. Thus, the changes in this population are most likely a secondary consequence of HIV-1 infection.

A poorly responsive immune system may result from an excess of suppression or a lack of induction. Much early work focused on the possibility that an excess of active suppression occurs in AIDS patients, and no substantial evidence for this has been found. Phenotypic subsets of CD8 T cells can be identified using two-color immunofluorescence. The cytotoxic subset (identified as CD11b-negative CD8 cells) tends to be elevated, and certain markers of activation/immaturity (Ia, CD38) that are elevated in AIDS occur within the CD8 compartment.[35,36] The relevance and relationships of these markers to pathogenesis and disease prognosis are not clearly understood.

Cytotoxic T-cell (CTL) responses to a specific virus, such as EBV, cytomegalovirus (CMV), and influenza also decline with progression of disease,[37–39] although it is not clear whether this results from a lack of CD4 help for the response or a loss of response by the CD8 cells themselves. In vitro, the virus does not inhibit the CD8 CTL response to EBV in normal individuals, although it is able to block the CD4 CTL response to another herpes virus, HSV-1.[40] This appears to result from a direct interaction between gp120 and CD4 on the effector cells, although a cell loss of CD4 CTL precursors could also play a role. Patients with AIDS often suffer from recurrent fulminating herpes lesions and also have an increased incidence of B-cell lymphomas. The loss of the CTL response that normally contain these viruses may explain these clinical findings.

Natural Killer Cells

Cells expressing NK-associated phenotypes and NK function tend to be well preserved in asymptomatic HIV-1-infected people but decline with advanced disease.[37] LGL or NK function in HIV-1 infection is of special interest for several reasons. Cells that are ordinarily resistant to NK lysis can be rendered susceptible by HIV-1 infection.[41] A subpopulation of LGL (lacking NK activity) have been shown to produce interferon alpha, which potentiates NK function and depresses HIV-1 replication in vitro.[42] The extent to which interferon alpha and NK function limit infection in vivo and whether preservation of these functions would prevent progression remain unknown.

B Cells

Hypergammaglobulinemia, elevated levels of immune complexes, and polyclonal B-cell activation are common findings in HIV-1-infected people. Although immunoglobulin levels are high, AIDS patients mount relatively poor antigen-specific antibody responses after vaccination. Primary responses are affected to a greater degree than secondary responses.[43] In asymptomatic people with HIV-1 infection who have not yet developed the immunodeficiency associated with severe clinical manifestations, antibody responses to vaccination tend to be normal, and no excess adverse reactions have been reported.[44]

The reason for polyclonal B-cell stimulation in HIV-1 infection remains an enigma. Several postulates have been put forth. In vitro, HIV-1 or HIV gp120 protein have been shown to polyclonally stimulate B cells either directly or indirectly through an action on T cells.[45] Epstein–Barr virus (EBV) is a polyclonal B-cell stimulator. Infection with EBV is almost universal in AIDS patients, and it is proposed that loss of T-cell control results in reactivation of latent EBV infection, leading to polyclonal

B-cell activation.[39] Other postulates for which there is less experimental support include a T-cell dysregulation phenomenon and the hypothesis that HIV-1-infected cells release B-cell-stimulating lymphokines.

Monocytes/Macrophages

Human monocytes and their tissue counterparts, macrophages, express the CD4 molecule and can be infected with HIV-1. HIV-1-infected monocytes appear to be the prime target of HIV-1 infection in the central nervous system.[5] Because monocytes replicate virus at low levels and do not die in vitro, it has been proposed that monocyte-derived cells are a more stable reservoir of infection than T cells. However, virus is inevitably detected in T cells from HIV-1-infected individuals by sensitive DNA amplification techniques and is only occasionally detected in monocytes.[46]

Many defects in monocyte function have been reported in HIV-1 infection. For the most part, these defects are inconsistently found and are more prominent in advanced disease. It is not clear whether the defects are a result of infection of monocytes, immunoregulatory T-cell imbalance, or supervening infections. For instance, the number of circulating monocytes is generally normal but may decline with advanced diseases. Similarly, defects in phagocytosis, intracellular killing, cytotoxicity, and class II MHC expression are most consistently found in patients with advanced disease. Antigen-specific proliferative responses are suppressed, and this is an early and relatively consistent feature of HIV infection.[33]

In vitro studies of anti-CD3-induced T-cell proliferation, which requires presentation of anti-CD3 by monocytes, have demonstrated a defect in presentation in monocytes from infected individuals.[47] Similarly, an HIV-infected monocytic cell line also shows impaired presentation in this system. However, defects in presentation of soluble antigen have yet to be convincingly demonstrated.

Natural History and Codeterminants of Progressive Disease

The natural history of HIV-1 infection is one of progressive CD4 T-cell depletion with increasing likelihood of clinical complications (Figure 4.1). Although perhaps intuitively expected, it has only recently been appreciated that progressive disease is associated with increased viral replication and viral burden in the chronically infected host.[48] Progressive CD4 T-cell depletion is a seemingly inexorable process related to duration of infection. However, there is clearly great heterogeneity in the rate at which infected people develop severe immunodeficiency. What determines this rate? In vitro studies of viral replication in acutely infected or latently

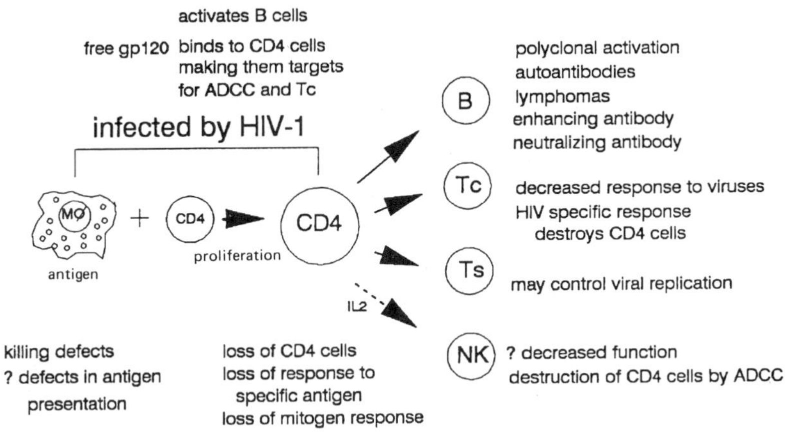

FIGURE 4.1. Immune dysfunction in HIV-1 infection.

infected cells clearly indicate that the activation state of the host cell is a major determinant of quantitative viral replication and cytopathicity.[6]

From these data, one might infer that cofactors that serve to activate T cells would hasten viral replication, T-cell depletion, and clinical deterioration. In clinical studies, it has been difficult to identify clinical, immunologic, or virologic features that predict progression. Features associated with progression have been described, but it has been difficult to determine whether they are simply a marker or consequence of severe immunodeficiency rather than a marker for a process that initiates progression. Markers reflecting a poor prognosis include low CD4 T cells (the best predictive marker), the onset of nonspecific symptoms (fever, weight loss), duration of infection, lower antibody titers to HIV-1, especially to the p24 core antigen, lower levels of antibodies that inhibit reverse transcriptase, elevated levels of p24 antigen, plasma viremia, higher in vivo titers of HIV-1, infection with or emergence of more virulent strains of HIV-1, elevated beta$_2$-microglobulin levels, and elevated levels of neopterin.[49]

Immune Response to HIV-1 Infection

People infected with HIV-1 mount and sustain a vigorous antibody response to HIV-1. Most people will generate detectable antibody within 3 months. Reports of prolonged seronegativity have been rare, difficult to confirm, and are controversial. With advanced immunodeficiency, antibody titers to most viral proteins diminish, with the curious, exception of antibody titers to the transmembrane protein, gp41.[50]

In established infection, it is not clear what role antibody plays in limiting infection nor is it clear how effective antibody would be if it were induced before infection (as by vaccination). Antibody titers decline with progressive disease, suggesting that high antibody levels maintain a stable, low level of infection. However, it is not clear whether declining antibody titers cause progression or are a consequence of it. Human anti-HIV-1 sera inevitably contain antibodies to the envelope protein. These inhibit virus binding to CD4 cells and have the capacity to neutralize infectivity.[51] They also mediate ADCC.[52] These same sera may contain antibodies that enhance infection in vitro.[53] Dissection of the antibody response has revealed antigenic determinants that elicit strain-specific and broadly neutralizing antibodies, that elicit T-cell responses, that are normally not immunogenic but potentially elicit a neutralizing response, and that have no apparent in vitro activity except possibly to interfere with binding by effective antibodies or perhaps mediate enhanced infection.[51,53–56] Obviously, the identification of relevant epitopes for induction of functionally important antibody responses is being actively investigated and is of paramount importance for vaccine development. The concept of protection by antibody is certainly feasible, because both passive and active immunization have met with limited success in animal models of retrovirus infection and, recently, in humans.[57,58]

For many viral diseases, antibody induced by vaccination or as a result of primary infection protects against infection on subsequent exposure, but it is the cellular response that is primarily responsible for resolution of infection. HIV-1 is unique in that the very cells that initiate a cellular response to HIV-1 are the cells destroyed by HIV-1. The sustained antibody response to HIV-1, which most certainly requires antigen-specific T/B collaboration, suggests that HIV-1-specific T cells do exist, and other observations previously discussed suggest that there may be phenotypic or functional immune profiles that indicate an attempt by the immune system to eliminate infection. Indeed, cellular responses to HIV-1 have been demonstrated. MHC-restricted, HIV-1-specific cytolytic CD8 T cells have been identified in HIV-1-infected people.[59] Noncytolytic CD8 T cells that inhibit viral replication or viral recovery in vitro have also been demonstrated.[60] The relationship to disease progression and the role in limiting infection of these cell-mediated responses have not yet been established.

Conclusion

The remarkable progress in research on HIV and the immune system has provided a solid foundation for understanding the molecular, cellular, and clinical pathogenesis of HIV-1 infection. HIV-1 has evolved an affinity for the CD4 molecule and a replication apparatus that is cytopathic for host cells: HIV-1 binds, penetrates, replicates in, and destroys CD4 T cells. Numerical/functional depletion of CD4 cells occurs over time, resulting in progressive paralysis of immune responsiveness and rendering the infected person susceptible to opportunistic infections and malignancies. Within this framework, much remains to be learned about factors that govern the control and extent of infection. The hope is that immunologic or other factors that control or prevent infection can be identified and applied successfully in this, as yet, incurable disease.

References

1. Fisher AG, Collalti E, Ratner L, Gallo RC, Wong-Stahl F. A molecular clone of HTLV-III with biological activity. Nature (London) 1985;316:262–265.
2. Levy JA, Cheng-Meyer C, Dina D, Luciw PA. AIDS retrovirus (ARV-2) clone replicates in transfected human and animal fibroblasts. Science 1986; 232:998–1000.
3. Srinivasan A, York D, Jannoun-Nasr R, Kalyanaraman V, Swan D, Benson J, Bohan C, Luciw P, Schnoll S, Robinson RA, Desai SM, Deuare SG. Generation of hybrid human immunodeficiency virus by homologous recombination. Proc Natl Acad Sci USA 1989;86:6388–6392.
4. Klatzman D, Barre-Sinoussi F, Nugeyre MT, Dauguet C, Vilmer E, Griscelli C, Brun-Vezinet F, Rouzioux C, Gluckman J-C, Chermann J-C, Montanier L. Selective tropism of lymphadenopathy-associated virus (LAV) for helper-inducer T lymphocytes. Science 1984;225:59–62.
5. Popovic M, Read-Connole E, Gallo R. T4 positive human neoplastic cell lines susceptible to and permissive for HTLV-III. Lancet 1984;ii:1472–1473.
6. McDougal JS, Mawle AC, Cort SP, Nicholson JKA, Cross GD, Scheppler-Campbell JA, Hicks D, Sligh J. Cellular tropism of the human retrovirus HTLV-III/LAV. I. Role of T cell activation and expression of the T4 antigen. J Immunol 1985;135:3151–3162.
7. Hoxie JA, Alpers JD, Rackowski JL, Huebner K, Haggary BS, Cedarbaum AJ, Reed JC. Alternations in T4 (CD4) protein and mRNA synthesis in cells infected with HIV. Science 1986;234:1123–1127.
8. Klatzmann D, Champagne E, Charmarat S, Gruest J, Guetard D, Hercend T, Gluckman J-C, Montagnier L. T-lymphocyte T4 molecule behaves as the receptor for human retrovirus LAV. Nature (London) 1985;312:767–768.
9. Dalgleish AG, Beverley PCL, Clapham PR, Crawford DH, Greaves MF, Weiss RA. The CD4 (T4) antigen is an essential component of the receptor for the AIDS retrovirus. Nature (London) 1985;312:763–767.
10. McDougal JS, Nicholson JKA, Cosand WL, Cross GD, Cort SP, Kennedy MS, Mawle AC. HIV binding to the CD4 molecule: conformation dependence and binding inhibition studies. In: D. Bolognesi, ed. Human Retroviruses, Cancer, and AIDS: Approaches to Prevention and Therapy. New York: Alan R. Liss, 1988;269–281.
11. McDougal JS, Kennedy MS, Sligh JM, Cort SP, Mawle A, Nicholson JKA. Binding of HLTV-III/LAV to $T4^+$ T cells by a complex of the 110K viral protein and the T4 molecule. Science 1986;231:382–385.
12. Maddon PJ, Dalgleish AG, McDougal JS, Clapham PR, Weiss RA, Axel R. The T4 gene encodes the AIDS virus receptor and is expressed in the immune system and in the brain. Cell 1986;47:333–348.

13. Clapham PR, Weber JV, Whitby D, McIntosh K, Dalgleish AG, Maddon PJ, Deen KC, Sweet RW, Weiss RA. Soluble CD4 blocks the infectivity of diverse strains of HIV and SIV for T cells but not for brain and muscle cells. Nature (London) 1989;337:368–370.
14. Nicholson JKA, Cross GD, Callaway CS, McDougal JS. In vitro infection of human monocytes with human T lymphotropic virus type III/lymphadenopathy-associated virus (HTLV-III/LAV). J Immunol 1986;137:323–329.
15. Gabudza DH, Ho DD, de la Monte SM, Hirsch MS, Rota TR, Sobel RA. Immunohistochemical identification of HTLV-III antigen in brains of patients with AIDS. Ann Neurol 1986;20:289–295.
16. Folks TM, Justement J, Kinter A, Dinarello CA, Fauci AS. Cytokine-induced expression of HIV-1 in a chronically infected promonocyte cell line. Science 1987;238:800–802.
17. Montagnier L, Gruest J, Chamaret S, Dauguet C, Axler C, Guetard D, Nugeyre MT, Barre-Sinoussi F, Chermann J-C. Adaptation of lymphadenopathy associated virus (LAV) to replication in EBV-transformed B lymphoblastoid cell lines. Science 1984;225:63–66.
18. Cheng-Mayer C, Rutka JT, Rosenblum ML, McHugh T, Stites DB, Levy JA. Human immunodeficiency virus can productively infect cultured glial cells. Proc Natl Acad Sci USA 1987;84:3526–3530.
19. DeRossi A, Franchinin G, Aldorini A, Del Mistro A, Chieco-Bianchi L, Gallo RC, Wong-Stahl F. Differential response to the cytopathic effects of human T-cell lymphotropic virus type III (HTLV-III) superinfection in $T4^+$ (helper) and $T8^+$ (suppressor) T cell clones transformed by HTLV-I. Proc Natl Acad Sci USA 1986;83:4297–4301.
20. Arthos J, Deen KC, Chaikin MA, Fornwald JA, Sathe G, Sattentau QJ, Clapham PR, Weiss RA, McDougal JS, Pietropaolo C, Axel R, Truneh A, Maddon PJ, Sweet RW. Identification of the residues in human CD4 critical for the binding of HIV. Cell 1989;57:469–481.
21. Lifson JD, Reyes GR, McGrath MS, Stein BS, Engleman EG. AIDS retrovirus induced cytopathology: giant cell formation and involvement of CD4 antigen. Science 1986;232:1123–1126.
22. Sodroski J, Goh WC, Rosen C, Campbell K, Haseltine WA. Role of the HTLV-III/LAV envelope in syncytium formation and cytopathicity. Nature 1986;322:470–474.
23. Lyerly HK, Matthews TJ, Langlois AS, Bolognesi DP, Weinhold KJ. Human T-cell lymphotropic virus III_B glycoprotein (gp120) bound to CD4 determinants on normal lymphocytes and expressed by infected cells serves as target for immune attack. Proc Natl Acad Sci USA 1987;84: 4601–4605.
24. Weinhold KJ, Lyerly HK, Matthews TJ, Tyler DS, Ahearne PM, Stine KC, Langlois AJ, Durack DT, Bolognesi DP. Cellular anti-gp120 cytolytic reactivities in HIV-1 seropositive individuals. Lancet 1988;i:902–905.
25. Siciliano RF, Lawton T, Knall C, Karr RW, Berman P, Gregory T, Reinherz EL. Analysis of host-virus interactions in AIDS with anti-gp120 T cell clones: effect of HIV sequence variation and a mechanism for $CD4^+$ cell depletion. Cell 1988;54:561–575.
26. Habeshaw JA, Dalgleish AG, Bountiff L, Newell AL, Wicks D, Walker LC, Manca F. 1990. AIDS pathogenesis: HIV envelope and its interactions with cell proteins. Immunol Today 1990;11:418–425.

27. Edelman AS, Zolla-Pazner S. AIDS: a syndrome of immune dysregulation, dysfunction, and deficiency. FASEB J 1989;3:22–30.
28. Nicholson JKA, McDougal JS, Spira TJ, Cross GD, Jones BM, Reinherz EL. Immunoregulatory subsets of the T helper and T suppressor cell population in homosexual men with chronic unexplained lymphadenopathy. J Clin Invest 1984;73:191–201.
29. Cooper DA, Gold J, Mallean P, Donovan B, Finlayson R, Barns TG, Michelmore HM, Brooke P, Penny R. Acute AIDS retrovirus infection: definition of a clinical illness associated with seroconversion. Lancet 1985; i:537–540.
30. Fahey JL, Prince H, Weaver MM, Groopman J, Visscher B, Schwartz K, Detels R. Quantitative changes in the Th or Ts lymphocyte subsets that distinguish AIDs syndromes from other immune subset disorders. Am J Med 1984;76:95–100.
31. Fauci AS, Macher H, Longo DL, Lane HC, Masur M, Gelman EP. Acquired immunodeficiency syndrome: epidemiological, clinical, immunologic and therapeutic considerations. Ann Intern Med 1984;100:92–106.
32. Wood GS, Burnes BF, Dorfman RD, Warnke RA. In situ quantitation of lymph node helper, suppressor, and cytotoxic T cell subsets in AIDS. Blood 1986;67:596–603.
33. Lane HC, Fauci AS. Immunological abnormalities in the acquired immunodeficiency syndrome. Annu Rev Immunol 1985;3:477–500.
34. Schnittman SM, Lane HC, Greenhouse J, Justement JS, Baseler M, Fauci AS. Preferential infection of $CD4^+$ memory cells by human immunodeficiency virus type 1: evidence for a role in the selective functional defects observed in infected individuals. Proc Natl Acad Sci USA 1990;87:6058–6062.
35. Nicholson JKA, Echenberg DF, Jones BM, Jaffe HW, Feorino PM, McDougal JS. T cytotoxic/suppressor cell phenotypes in a group of asymptomatic homosexual men with and without exposure to HTLV-III/LAV. Clin Immunol Immunopathol 1986;40:505–514.
36. Salazar-Gonzalez JF, Moody DJ, Giorgi JV, Martinez-Maza O, Mitsuyasu RT, Fahey JL. Reduced ecto-5′ nucleotidase activity and enhanced OKT10 and HLA-DR expression on CD8 (T suppressor/cytotoxic) lymphocytes in the acquired immune deficiency syndrome: evidence of CD8 immaturity. J Immunol 1985;135:1778–1785.
37. Rook AH, Manischewitz JF, Frederick WR, Epstein JS, Jackson L, Gelman E, Steis R, Masur H, Quinnan GV. Deficient HLA-restricted cytomegalovirus-specific cytotoxic T cells and natural killer cells in patients with the acquired immune deficiency syndrome. J Infect Dis 1985;152:627–630.
38. Shearer GM, Salahuddin SZ, Markham PD, Joseph LJ, Payne SM, Kriebel P, Bernstein DC, Biddison WE, Sarngadharan MG, Gallo RC. Prospective study of cytotoxic T lymphocyte responses to influenza and antibodies to human lymphotrophic virus-III in homosexual men. J Clin Invest 76: 1699–1704.
39. Birx DL, Redfield RR, Tosato R. Defective regulation of Epstein–Barr virus infection in patients with acquired immune deficiency syndrome or AIDS-related disorders. N Engl J Med 1986;314:874–879.
40. Mawle AC, Thieme ML, Ridgeway MR, McDougal JS, Schmid DS. Inhibition of the in vitro generation of class II-restricted, HSV-1-specific $CD4^+$ CTL by HIV-1. AIDS Res Hum Retrovir 1990;6:229–241.

41. Ruscetti FW, Mikouits JA, Kalyanaraman VS, Overton R, Stevenson H, Stromberg K, Herberman RB, Farrar WL, Ortaldo JR. Analysis of effector mechanisms against HTLV-1 and HTLV-III/LAV infected lymphoid cells. J Immunol 1986;136:3619–3624.
42. Ho DD, Hartshorn KL, Rota TR, Andrews C, Kaplan JC, Schooley R, Hirsch MS. Recombinant human interferon alpha-A suppresses HTLV-III replication in vitro. Lancet 1985;i:602–604.
43. Lane HC, Masur H, Edgar LC, Whalen G, Rook AH, Fauci AS. Abnormalities of B cell activation and immunoregulation in patients with the acquired immunodeficiency syndrome. N Engl J Med 1983;309:453–458.
44. Huang KL, Ruben FL, Rinaldo CR, Kingsley L, Lyter DW, Ho M. Antibody responses after influenza and pneumococcal immunization in HIV-infected homosexual men. JAMA 1987;257:2047–2050.
45. Schnittman SM, Lane HC, Higgins SE, Folks T, Fauci AS. Direct polyclonal activation of human B lymphocytes by the acquired immune deficiency virus. Science 1986;233:1084–1086.
46. Meltzer MS, Skillman DR, Hoover DL, Hanson BD, Turpan JA, Kalter DC, Gendelman HE. Macrophages and the human immunodeficiency virus. Immunol Today 1990;11:217–223.
47. Prince HE, Moody DJ, Shubin BI, Fahey JF. Defective monocyte function in acquired immune deficiency syndrome (AIDS): evidence from a monocyte-dependent proliferative system. J Clin Invest 1985;5:21–25.
48. Nicholson JKA, Spira TJ, Aloisio CH, Jones BM, Kennedy MS, Holman RC, McDougal JS. Serial determinations of HIV-1 titers in HIV-infected homosexual men: association of rising titers with CD4 T cell depletion and progression to AIDS. AIDS Res Hum Retrovir 1989;5:205–215.
49. Hessol NA, Lifson AR, Rutherford GW. Natural history of human immunodeficiency virus and key predictors of disease progression. In: P Volberding, MA Jacobson, eds. AIDS Clinical Reviews. M. Dekker, New York, 1989: 69–93.
50. Sarngadharan MG, Popovic M, Bruch L, Schupbach J, Gallo RC. Antibodies reactive with human T-lymphotropic retroviruses (HTLV-III) in the serum of patients with AIDS. Science 1984;224:506–508.
51. Looney DJ, Fisher AG, Putney SD, Rusche JR, Redfield RR, Burke DS, Gallo RC, Wong-Stahl F. Type-restricted neutralization of molecular clones of human immunodeficiency virus. Science 1988;241:357–359.
52. Ojo-Amaize EA, Mishanian P, Keith DE, Houghton RL, Heitjan DF, Fahey JL, Giorgi JV. Antibodies to human immunodeficiency virus induce cell-mediated lysis of human immunodeficiency virus-infected cells. J Immunol 1987;139:2458–2463.
53. Matsuda S, Gidlund M, Chiodi F, Cafaro A, Nygren A, Morein B, Fenyo E-M, Wigzel H. Enhancement of human immunodeficiency virus (HIV) replication in human monocytes by low titers of anti-HIV antibodies in vitro. Scand J Immunol 1989;30:425–434.
54. Ho DD, Sarngadharan MG, Hirsch MS, Schooley RT, Rota TR, Kennedy RC, Chanh TC, Sato VL. Human immunodeficiency virus neutralizing antibodies recognize several conserved domains on the envelope glycoproteins. J Virol 1987;61:2024–2028.

55. Weiss RA, Clapham PR, Weber NJ, Dalgleish AG, Lasky LA, Berman PW. Variable and conserved neutralization antigens of human immunodeficiency virus. Nature (London) 1986;324:572–575.
56. Krohn K, Robey WG, Putney S, Arthur L, Nara P, Fischinger P, Gallo RC, Wong-Stahl F, Ranki A. Specific cellular immune response and neutralizing antibodies in goats immunized with native or recombinant envelope proteins derived from human T-lymphotropic virus type III_{β} and in human immunodeficiency virus-infected men. Proc Natl Acad Sci USA 1987;84:4994–4998.
57. Murphy-Corb M, Martin LN, Davison-Fairburn B, Montelaro RC, Miller M, West M, Ohkawa S, Baskin GB, Zhang JY, Putney SD, Allison AC, Eppstein DA. A formalin-inactivated whole SIV vaccine confers protection in macaques. Science 1989;246:1293–1297.
58. Karpas A, Hewlett IK, Hill F, Gray J, Byrom N, Gilgen D, Bally V, Oates JK, Gazzard B, Epstein JE. Polymerase chain reaction evidence for human immunodeficiency virus 1 neutralization by passive immunization in patients with AIDS and AIDS-related complex. Proc Natl Acad Sci USA 1990;87: 7613–7617.
59. Walker BD, Plata F. Cytotoxic T lymphocytes against HIV. AIDS 1990; 4:177–184.
60. Walker CM, Moody DJ, Stites DP, Levy JA. $CD8^+$ T lymphocyte control of HIV replication in cultured $CD4^+$ cells varies among infected individuals. Cell Immunol 1989;119:470–475.

5
Serologic Tests for the Detection of Human Immunodeficiency Virus Infection

J. RICHARD GEORGE and GERALD SCHOCHETMAN

Persons infected with the human immunodeficiency virus (HIV) have a spectrum of clinical features, ranging from persons who are infected but appear completely healthy to those with rapid disease progression and mortality. All groups, regardless of clinical stage, possess several biologic indicators of viral infection or replication (Figure 5.1). These include viremia, antibodies against viral proteins, circulating viral proteins, and nonspecific markers such as neopterin, beta$_2$-microglobulins, and T_4 cell counts. A variety of immunologic tests currently exists for the detection of viral antibodies and protein antigens. These assays have permitted testing programs to protect the blood supply from infected units and to conduct seroprevalence surveys to define the epidemic. More recently, the presence or absence of viral and nonspecific markers have been used to predict the onset of clinical disease.

Of the tests available for HIV diagnosis (Table 5.1), enzyme immunoassays (EIA) or enzyme-linked immunosorbent assays (ELISA) for HIV-1 antibody are the most widely used. They provide a low-cost, effective screening test for HIV-1 infection. To date, the U.S. Food and Drug Administration (FDA) has licensed 10 EIA tests for HIV-1 antibody; however, 1 test is no longer in production. When properly used, sera are screened by EIA using a single determination. Specimens found to be nonreactive are reported as negative. Specimens that are reactive by the initial EIA are retested in duplicate. If either of the duplicate tests is positive, the sera are said to be repeatedly reactive and must then be tested by a supplemental assay, such as immunofluorescence (IFA) or western blot.[1–4] Patients are informed that they are positive only when they are repeatedly reactive by EIA and are IFA or western blot positive. Results from the EIA alone should never be reported.

Use of trade names is for identification only and does not constitute endorsement by the Public Health Service or the the U.S. Department of Health and Human Services.

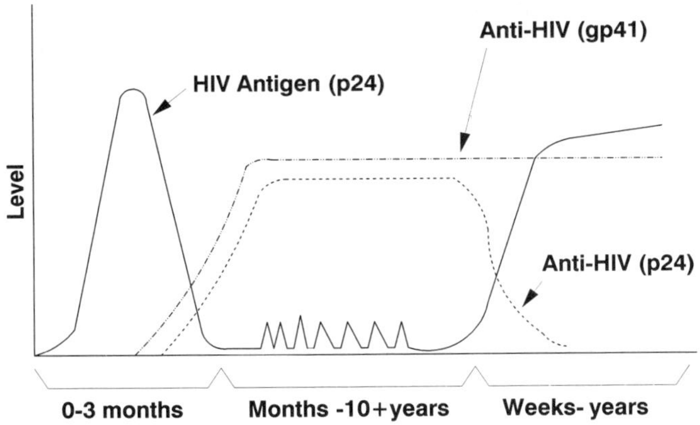

FIGURE 5.1. Natural history of HIV-1 infections.

Enzyme Immunoassay for HIV Antibody Detection

In 1985, the first five HIV-1 antibody kits were licensed by the FDA. Since that time, HIV testing for diagnosis and seroprevalence in the United States has been based on the use of these kits. Then, in 1987, the first confirmed case of HIV-2 was found in the United States.[5] Subsequently, a total of 21 additional cases have been confirmed, all from

TABLE 5.1. Tests for detection of HIV infections.

ANTIBODY TESTS
Enzyme immunoassays (EIA)
Whole virus lysate antigens
Recombinant protein antigens
Chemically synthesized antigens
Other types of screening assays
Particle agglutination assays
Hemaaaglutination assays
Latex agglutination assays
Solid-phase immunoassays
Supplemental tests
Immunoblotting (western blot)
Immunofluorescence assay (IFA)
Radioimmunoprecipitation assay (RIPA)
Virus neutralization
TESTS FOR VIRUS OR VIRAL ANTIGENS
Enzyme immunoassays (antigen capture)
Radioimmunoassay
Antigen capture
Competitive inhibition
Virus culture

individuals who had recently migrated from or visited West Africa.[6] In 1989, the first U.S. native infected with HIV-2 was identified in the northeastern United States.[7] These discoveries led to a reevaluation of the need to screen blood donations for HIV-2 in the United States and to expand HIV-2 serosurveys. Currently, most blood collection centers rely on the cross-reactivity between HIV-1 EIAs for HIV-2 antibodies to detect HIV-2-infected units. HIV-1 EIAs have bveen found to detect between 9% and 91.0% of HIV-2-infected specimens.[8,9] Obviously, there is a chance that infected units could be missed using this approach. Therefore, it became necessary to develop independent tests for HIV-2 antibody. The first of these kits was licensed in April 1990.

Several companies have similar tests under development using either recombinant or chemically synthesized antigens. Most experts believe that future assays will be combination assays that simultaneously detect HIV-1 and HIV-2 antibodies in a single well. These combination tests are proving to be quite popular in Europe where HIV-2 testing is more common.[10,11] Because of the low prevalence of HIV-2 in the United States, the FDA has not yet mandated that the blood supply be screened for this virus. However, if the situation in the United States parallels that of Europe, testing for HIV-2 may eventually be necessary. Several U.S. blood collection centers have begun voluntary screening with HIV-2-specific EIAs.

Commercial enzyme immunoassays for HIV-1 and HIV-2 antibody use several types of antigens, that is, whole virus lysate, recombinant proteins, and chemically synthesized peptides. The first FDA-approved assays using a whole virus lysate antigen[12] remain the most commonly used antigen

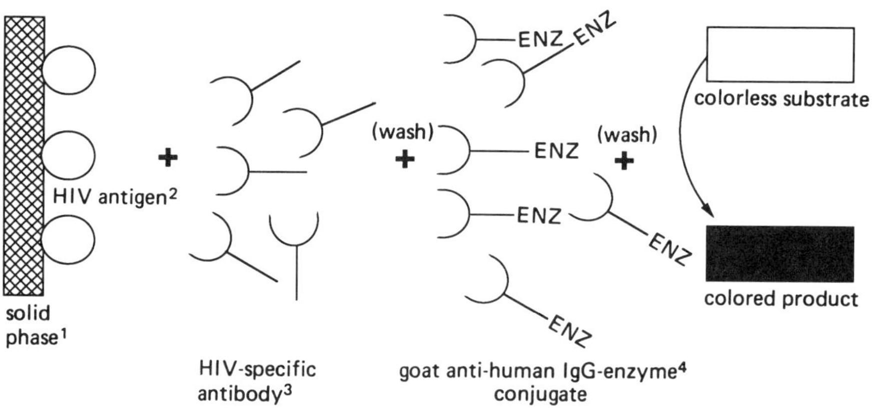

FIGURE 5.2. Configuration of enzyme-linked immunosorbent assay (ELISA), or indirect enzyme immunoassay (EIA), for antibodies against HIV. Key: 1, microplate well or other surface; 2, whole virus lysate, recombinant, or chemically synthesized; 3, patient's serum or plasma; 4, horseradish peroxidase or alkaline phosphatase.

preparation in the United States. These assays are thought to be more sensitive than EIAs using fewer recombinant or chemically synthesized antigens, because whole virus lysate antigens contain all the viral proteins present in the virus. On the other hand, they also contain proteins from the cells used to grow the virus as well as from the cell culture medium. Therefore, these assays tend to be less specific than assays based on recombinant or synthetic antigens.

Enzyme immunoassays for HIV antibodies can be configured in a variety of ways, the most common of which is the indirect assay (Figure 5.2). The viral, synthetic, or recombinant antigens are bound to a solid support, and the patient's serum or plasma is incubated with the fixed antigens. If any of the antibodies (immunoglobulins) bind to the antigens, this will be detected when an antihuman immunoglobulin G (IgG) antibody is added. The antihuman IgG is labeled by conjugation with an enzyme (e.g., alkaline phosphatase or horseradish peroxidase) so that when a substrate is added an enzymatic reaction will produce a color reaction of an intensity proportional to the amount of human antibody to HIV present.

The competitive assay is a second method of configuring an EIA for the detection of HIV antibody (Figure 5.3). Competitive assays use the same types of antigens as the indirect EIA. These antigens are bound to a solid support, usually a plastic microplate well. The patient's sample (serum or plasma) is added to the well simultaneously with enzyme-labeled HIV antibody. For competitive assays to be accurate and precise, the same amount of antigen and conjugated antibody must be present in every

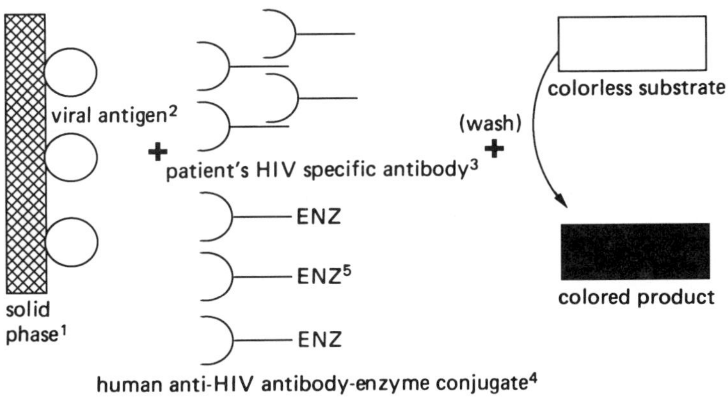

FIGURE 5.3. Configuration of competitive enzyme immunoassay for antibodies against HIV. Key: 1, microplate well or other surface; 2, whole virus lysate, recombinant, or chemically synthesized; 3, patient's serum or plasma; 4, human polyclonol or monoclonal, quantity limited and fixed (added simultaneously with 3); 5, horseradish peroxidase or alkaline phosphatase.

well. Usually the amount of conjugated antibody added is sufficient to saturate available antigen binding sites. During incubation, the patient's antibodies compete with the enzyme-labeled antibody for the limited number of antigen binding sites available on the walls of the microplate. If there are no HIV antibodies present in the sample, all antigen binding sites are occupied by enzyme-labeled antibody and after incubation with substrate give the maximum possible absorbance. As the concentration of antibody increases in the patient's sample, the enzyme-labeled antibody is displaced from the antigen binding site and the color development is less than observed with antibody-negative specimens. In contrast to the indirect assays, the intensity of the color change observed in the competitive EIA is inversely related to the amount of HIV antibody present in the test sample.

The sensitivity and specificity of commercial EIAs were found to be between 98.1% and 100.0% in a study that compared their results to western blot.[13] It has been estimated that when properly performed, the average specificity of EIA tests is 99.8.[3] In routine blood bank practice, currently 0.21–0.66% of samples are initially reactive and 0.03–0.33% are repeatedly reactive.[14] The percentage of repeatedly reactive specimens found to be positive by supplemental tests varies according to the true antibody prevalence of the tested population. As a national average, the prevalence of western blot-positive samples among blood donors has been estimated to be 0.017%.[14]

While commercial EIA tests are very sensitive, it should be noted that false-negative results may occur. Seroconversion usually occurs 2 to 3 months after exposure to the virus[15–20] but may not occur for 5 months[21] or longer if the individual is immunocompromised.[22] FDA-licensed EIAs and western blots primarily detect IgG antibody to HIV and would be negative in early infections before the switch from IgM to IgG antibody.[23,24] This switch has been reported to take as long as 41 weeks.[23,25] Tests to detect these antibodies are discussed later in this chapter.

False-positive EIAs do occur and can cause considerable anxiety if these results are reported before performing a supplemental test. In general, the probability of an EIA-positive result being false positive is inversely related to the intensity of the reaction. In a low-prevalence population (volunteer blood donors), 86.7% of the strongly reactive EIA results were also western blot or culture positive. On the other hand, sera that were EIA weakly or moderately reactive were western blot or culture positive only 1.9% of the time.[26] False-positive EIA results have been attributed to a number of conditions and practices. False-positive results may result from the intrinsic variation of EIA tests, which has been estimated to be as great as 13.0% for antibody levels close to the cutoff.

Heat-treated, lipemic, and hemolyzed sera have also been implicated in false-positivity. HLA antibodies with specificity for HLA DQ3 and HLA

DR4 antigens (found in H-9 cell lines used in the production of viral antigen) and probably other contaminating antigens from cell lines[27,28] can also cause the EIA test to be positive. False-positive results have also been found to occur in 19% of hemophilia patients,[29] 13% of alcoholic patients with hepatitis,[30] 4% of hemodialysis patients,[31] and 24% of patients with a positive rapid reagin test.[32] For these reasons, and because of the considerable psychologic and social implications of being HIV antibody positive, it is inappropriate either to counsel people or to make medical decisions about them based on EIA testing alone. Persons who are initially reactive by EIA are retested in duplicate. Repeatedly reactive specimens are then tested with a supplemental tests such as IFA or western blot before test results are revealed to the patient.

Other Screening Assays

Agglutination Assays

Other than EIA, the particle agglutination assay SERODIA-HIV (Fujirebio Inc., Japan) is the most widely used screening test for HIV antibody. Because this test has not been licensed by the FDA, it is more widely used in Asia, Australia, South America, and Africa. The assay is simpler to perform than the standard EIA and requires practically no equipment (Figure 5.4). The assay is, however, well suited for use in large seroprevalence surveys. It is performed by mixing 25 μl of a diluted serum with a suspension of gelatin particles coated with purified HIV antigen. The

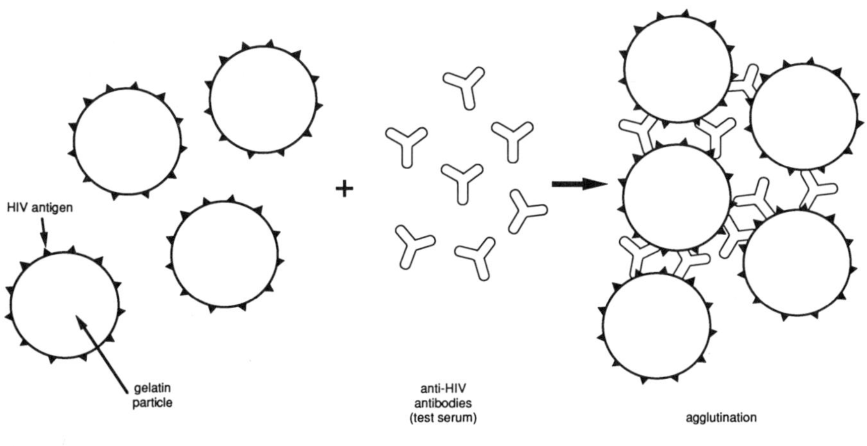

FIGURE 5.4. All agglutination tests have essentially the same mechanism. Particles such as gelatin (shown) or latex are coated with viral antigen. In the presence of HIV antibody, particles are cross-linked and agglutination occurs.

assay is performed in a microplate and can be read after incubating for 2 hours at room temperature. Sera that agglutinate coated particles alone are read as positive; sera that produce no agglutination are negative; sera that agglutinate both coated and uncoated particles are retested after absorption with a suspension of uncoated particles. Positive specimens should be confirmed by the use of a supplemental assay such as western blot.

The particle agglutination assay has been found to be slightly less sensitive[33,34] and less specific[33–35] than EIA. However, the differences were not large and with some specimens (early seroconverters) the assay was more sensitive. This was thought to be because of the presence of IgM or IgA antibodies being detected by the agglutination assay and missed by the IgG-specific EIA tests. Samples that often gave false-positive results by EIA, including heat-treated specimens, specimens containing HLA antibodies, specimens containing autoantibodies, and specimens from individuals with a history of multiple blood transfusions, were found to be negative by particle agglutination.[35]

A second agglutination test, Recombigen HIV Latex Agglutination assay, has been licensed by the FDA for use as a screening assay. This assay has not gained wide acceptance because of its cost, difficulty in reading, and lack of sensitivity (95.2%) and specificity (96.1%) as compared to EIA.[33] The assay is very easy to perform and produces results in less than 10 minutes. However, it is difficult to read even when the appropriate high-intensity light and magnification are used as recommended by the manufacturer. When performed by well-trained, experienced technologists the results have been found to be reliable.[36]

A passive agglutination test (Quick PHT-HIV, Salck Industries, Sao Paulo, Brazil) has seen limited use in laboratories outside of Brazil. This assay is intended for use in the same situations as a the SERODIA-HIV particle agglutination tests, and the methodology is very similar. However, the Salck test has been found to be very insensitive and less specific than SERODIA-HIV.[37]

Other Rapid Tests

Several solid-phase EIAs in which HIV antigens (whole virus lysate, recombinant, or synthetic) are immobilized on a membrane (HIV-CHEK, Du Pont, Wilmington, Delaware; Abbott Test Pack HIV-1/2, Abbott Park, Illinois; and Genie 1/2, Seattle, Washington) are in use in many laboratories around the world. These assays are often referred to as "rapid tests" because results can be obtained in 10–15 minutes. However, none of the tests have yet been licensed in the United States. The antigens are reacted with the patient's sera, and the resulting immune complexes are trapped onto filters. Subsequent detection of immune complexes is accomplished by the sequential reaction with enzyme–

antihuman IgG conjugates and then a precipitating substrate. A color reaction develops at the site where immune complexes are present and stains the membrane. The tests are read as positive or negative on the basis of the presence of the color reaction as compared to positive and negative control spots.

These assays have been gaining in popularity because they are simple and provide rapid results. They are targeted for situations in which

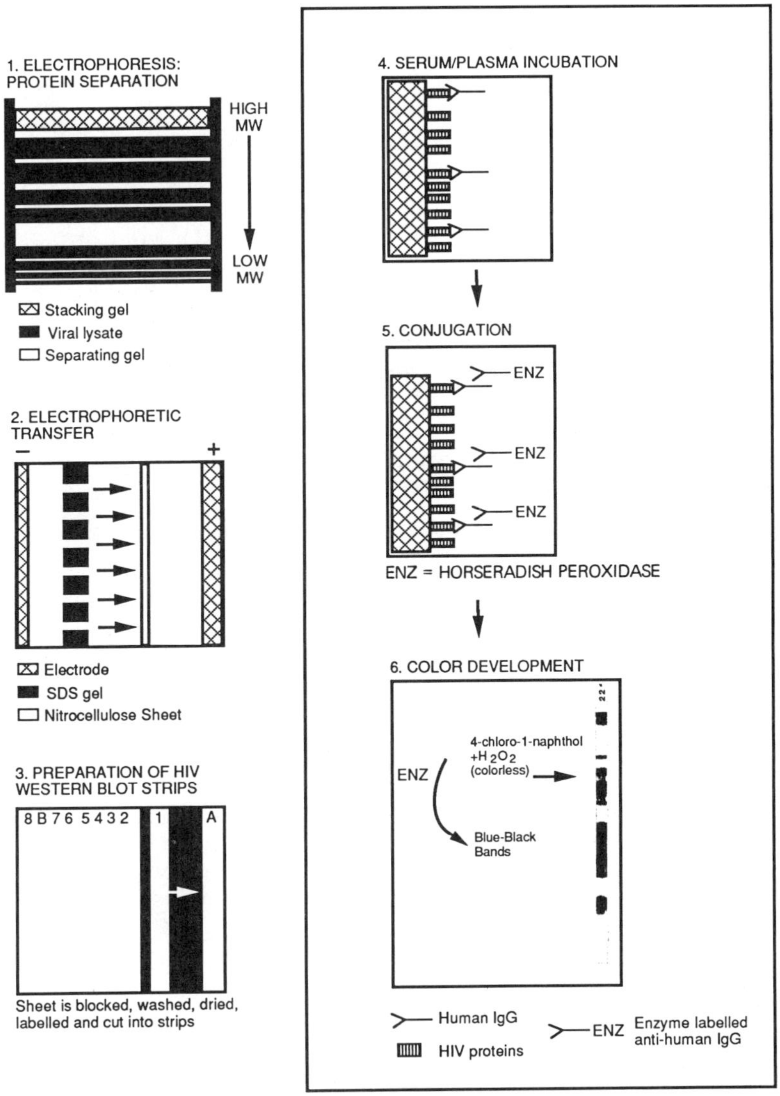

FIGURE 5.5. Step-by-step performance of western blot supplemental test for antibodies against HIV.

standard EIAs cannot be performed or immediate test results are required. Their use in developing nations has been limited because they cost more ($2–$10 per test) than the EIA (<$1). However, as with EIAs, they produce false-positive results and must be confirmed by a supplemental test before notifying the patient of the results. Most of these tests are new, and few data are available on their performance. However, published reports have found HIV-CHEK to be 95% sensitive and 99% specific[37,38]; the GENIE 1/2 is 99.8% sensitive and 95% specific.[39]

Western Blot

The western blot (WB) assay[40] is a more informative followup test for EIA. The WB uses separated HIV proteins immobilized on nitrocellulose paper to determine which antibodies in the sample are responsible for the reactivity observed in the EIA. Partially purified HIV viral proteins are fractionated according to their molecular weight by electrophoresis on a polyacrylamide separating gel (Figure 5.5). The smaller, lower molecular weight proteins are able to move through the gel more readily than the larger, high molecular weight proteins and migrate to the bottom of the gel.

A sheet of nitrocellulose is next applied to the surface of the gel. An electric current is applied, causing the proteins to migrate from the gel to the surface of the nitrocellulose. After blocking and washing, the nitro-

TABLE 5.2 Identification of major structural gene products of HIV-1 and HIV-2 by their molecular weight in western blot and their recommended nomenclature.

Gene	Gene product	HIV-1 nomenclature	Gene product	HIV-2 nomenclature
ENV	gp160	Precursor[a]		
	gp120	External envelope	gp125[b]	External envelope
	gp41	Transmembrane	gp36/41[c]	Transmembrane
			gp70[d]	Dimeric form of Transmembrane
POL	p66	Reverse transcriptase	p68	Reverse transcriptase
	p51	Reverse transcriptase	p56	Reverse transcriptase
	p32	Endonuclease	p55	Reverse transcriptase
			p34	Endonuclease
GAG	p55	Precursor		
	p40	Precursor		
	p24	Core	p26	Core
	p17	Matrix	p16	Matrix

[a] Usually not present. Often confused with oligomeric form of gp41.
[b] Identified as gp105 by some manufacturers. Usually present but often obscured by oligomeric forms of transmembrane glycoprotein.
[c] Different virus strains may produce one or both forms of transmembrane glycoprotein.
[d] Sometimes seen on some commercial reagents.

cellulose page is cut into strips. An appropriate dilution of serum or plasma found to be repeatedly reactive on an HIV EIA is incubated with a strip. Human antibodies to HIV proteins, if present, will bind to the viral antigens bound to the surface of the nitrocellulose. After washing off unbound materials, the strips are incubated with goat antibody against human IgG that has been conjugated with an enzyme, either horseradish peroxidase or alkaline phosphatase. If antibody is bound during the initial incubation, the conjugate will bind to the immune complex. In the final step, an appropriate substrate is added to the strip. Following conversion of the colorless substrate by enzyme, colored bands will appear wherever human IgG was bound to proteins on the strip. The identity and position of these proteins are established by comparison to a standard sera known to react with all the viral bands listed in Table 5.2 and shown in Figure 5.6.

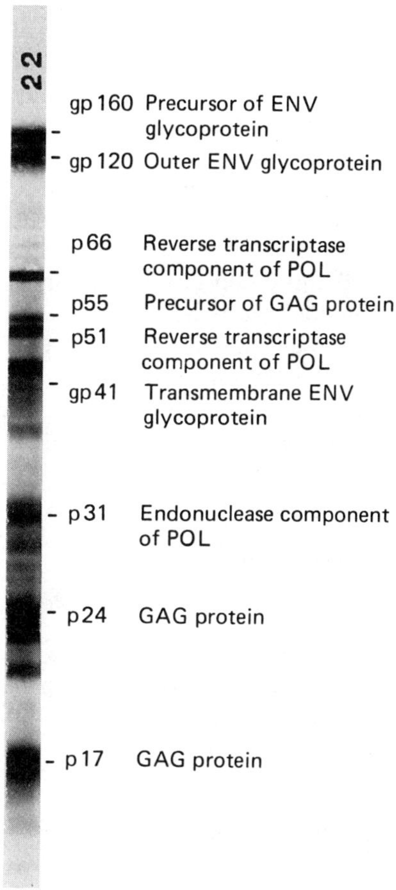

FIGURE 5.6. Major structural proteins seen on HIV-1 western blot.

Interpretion of western blot tests relies on the structural proteins coded for by the *env*, *pol*, and *gag* genes (Table 5.2). Most reports indicate that antibodies to *gag* proteins appear first on the western blot test. For HIV-1 infections, these antibodies appear to decrease or become undetectable with the onset of clinical symptoms.[40–45] In contrast, antibodies to the external glycoprotein and the transmembrane proteins can be detected in nearly all HIV-1-infected patients regardless of clinical stage.[46–48] Antibodies to the *pol* gene product are often detected if the antigens are present on the strips. Their diagnostic value is low compared to the *gag* and *env* proteins. Antibodies against other HIV proteins *tat*, *vif*, *nef*, and other *gag* proteins are detected less often and are not routinely used as markers of infection.

It is interesting to note that considerable confusion remains over the accurate identification of *env* glycoproteins present on commercial HIV-1 and HIV-2 western blots. Recent reports regarding HIV-1 western blots[49,50] have reported that a number of commercial western blots misidentified the 120-kd and 160-kd bands on their strips as representing the external glycoprotein and the envelope precursor glycoprotein, respectively. In fact, these bands represented trimeric and tetrameric forms of the transmembrane glycoprotein (TMP), gp41. These studies showed that the true precursor and external glycoproteins were not present on most commercial western blots. On those strips where the external envelope was present, it banded at the same position as the trimeric form of the TMP and could not be distinquished from this glycoprotein.

Similar observations have been made for the glycoproteins of HIV-2 (Figure 5.7). The TMP of HIV-2 was found to exist as a full-length glycoprotein (gp41) in some isolates and in a truncated form (gp36) in others. Some isolates can produce both forms. Studies have shown that both forms of the TMP often are present on commercial western blots as

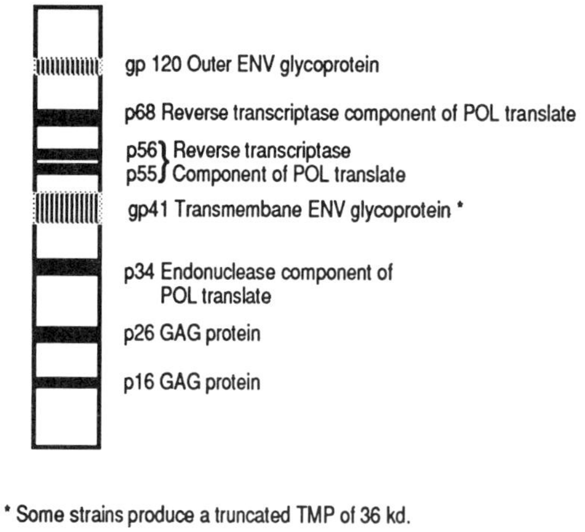

FIGURE 5.7. Major structural proteins seen on HIV-2 western blot.

trimers, again binding at the same position as the external glycoprotein. The envelope precursor has not been found to be present at significant levels in commercial western blots for HIV-1 or HIV-2. This often leads to misinterpretation by existing interpretive criteria and precludes the correct identification of antibodies to the viral glycoproteins.

Despite the overall sensitivity and specificity of western blots there has been extensive debate over the best interpretive criteria. This debate increased when it was found that considerable cross-reactivity exists between HIV-1 and HIV-2 antibodies by western blot.[51] This has been found to be especially true in West African countries centering around Cote d'Ivoire. Cross-reactivity between antibodies against *gag* and *pol* is expected and was predicted based on the sequence homology that exists for HIV-1 and HIV-2. It was, however, somewhat surprising to discover that extensive cross-reactivity occurred between the *env* transmembrane glycoprotein. In a study of 1362 consecutive tuberculosis (TB) patients and 2127 consecutive blood donors in Abidjan, Cote d'Ivoire, it was found that 73% and 83%, respectively, of all EIA positives were dually reactive by western blot.[51] Efforts to classify infections as HIV-1 or HIV-2 has had considerable influence on the selection of interpretive criteria for HIV-1 and especially for HIV-2.

Various interpretive criteria for HIV-1 and HIV-2 are presented in Table 5.3. In the United States, the Centers for Disease Control/Association of State and Territorial Public Health Laboratory Directors (CDC/ASTPHLD) criteria[53] is the most frequently applied standard. A serum is interpreted as positive by this standard when two of the bands p24, gp41, or gp120/gp160 are present. A negative test interpretation requires the absence of all bands. Any other pattern is regarded as indeterminate. As presented in Table 5.3, several other groups have presented interpretive criteria. Some such as the Ortho/Du Pont FDA-approved western blot recommend very conservative criteria. These criteria interpret sera as positive when bands detected include p24, p31, and either a diffuse gp41 or gp120/160 band. This strict interpretation maximizes the specificity of the test and is mainly intended for use with samples from individuals at low risk of HIV infection, such as blood donors, for whom there is no other clinical information. These criteria may not be suited for all situations, especially the testing of persons at increased risk or with symptoms suggestive of HIV infection. Criteria that require the presence of *gag*, *pol*, and *env* gene products for a positive interpretation to be made have a reduced sensitivity for diagnosis in AIDS patients who may have already lost their *gag*/*pol* antibodies.[45,53]

The diagnosis of HIV-2 infection by western blot is based heavily on the specific and sensitive detection of antibodies to the *env* glycoproteins.[54] This definition classifies a patient as HIV-2 infected on the basis of the presence of two glycoprotein bands (gp36/41, gp105, or gp140). Unfortunately, this interpretation is based on the misidentified *env* glycopro-

TABLE 5.3. Criteria for positive interpretation of western blot tests.

Organization	Criteria for HIV-1	Criteria for HIV-2
Organization of State and Territorial Public Health Laboratory Directors/CDC	Any two of: p24 gp41 gp120/160	None
FDA-licensed Biotech/ DuPont Test	p24 and p31 and gp41 or gp120/160	None
American Red Cross	One band from each gene-product group (total of 3): *gag* and *pol* and *env*	None
Consortium for Retrovirus Serology Standardization	Two or more bands: p24 or p31 plus gp41 or gp120/160	None
World Health Organization[a]	Two *env* bands with or without *gag* or *pol*	Two *env* bands with or without *gag* or *pol*

[a] All criteria, except WHO, score blots with no bands as **NEGATIVE**. WHO scores blots as **NEGATIVE** if bands are present that do not correspond to the structural proteins listed in Table 5.2. All other patterns not scored as positive are **INDETERMINATE**.

teins, as previously discussed. It would appear that the best criteria would be based on the presence of *gag* (p26) and/or *pol* (p34) and the transmembrane glycoprotein (gp36/41). The additional presence of the external glycoprotein (gp120) would be supporting evidence of HIV-2 infection, but because of the strain specificity observed this should not be mandatory for a positive interpretation.

In a large clinical study involving screening of a low-risk population, it has been estimated that the false-positive rate of combined EIA and western blot testing is less than 1:100,000.[55]

Indeterminate or "atypical" western blot patterns occur much more frequently and cause greater concern than false-positive results. Indeterminate patterns (e.g., p17 or p24 only) can occur in as many as 15% of samples tested by the western blot, and despite recommendations to the contrary, many uninfected persons may be told that they have an indeterminate result without a clear explanation of its meaning. Cumulative experience from nearly 5 years of testing suggests that indeterminate western blot patterns that do not change for many months or years do not indicate HIV infection.[56–58] Persons with persistently indeterminate western blot patterns usually do not have risk factors for HIV infection, do not manifest laboratory signs of immunodeficiency, and do not develop disease states typical of HIV infection. However, virologic data on long-term followup of persistently indeterminate cohorts were not available until recently.

Two recent studies[59,60] have followed populations of blood donors with persistently indeterminate (>6 months) HIV-1 western blot results up to 2 years and found them to be free of HIV infection. It was shown that none of these uninfected blood donors had detectable HIV proviral DNA when analyzed by polymerase chain reaction (PCR) technique or by culture for HIV-1. On the basis of these results, it is clear that persons having persistent indeterminate western blots should be counseled that they should continue to monitor the band pattern by western blot for at least 6 months; if no additional bands develop, they should then be advised that they are negative for HIV-1 infection.

Blood donors who are repeatedly EIA reactive but are negative by supplemental tests are most likely not infected.[61] However, blood donated by these individuals should not be used for transfusion unless the donors are subsequently found to be negative by both EIA and a licensed western blot on two separate occasions at least 6 months apart. There is an extremely low probability that EIA-positive, western blot-negative individuals from low-risk groups are HIV infected. Therefore, it is not recommended that they be notified of their "false-positive" EIA result. However, this practice is objectionable to some blood banks who think it is less ethical not to inform the donors and to continue drawing units that are discarded.

Immunofluorescence Assay

Many laboratories find the western blot tests to be too expensive for use in high-volume situations. This is especially true in developing nations where the additional problem of availability of western blot must be considered. The immunofluorescence assay (IFA) offers a low-cost alternative as a supplemental assay.[62–67] Many laboratories using this procedure prepare their own reagents. Typically, lymphocytes infected with HIV are inactivated and fixed in acetone on glass slides. Uninfected cells of the same line are either mixed with the infected cells or placed on a separate area of the slide to serve as negative controls. Serum dilutions are incubated with cell preparations, washed, and then incubated with fluorescein isothiocyanate-labeled anti-human IgG. Positive and negative control sera should be included on each slide. Antibodies in the positive sera bind to the viral antigens expressed by the infected cells. A test is interpreted as positive on the basis of the percentage of fluorescent cells and the type of fluorescence patterns observed (peripheral versus cytoplasmic staining). The reports previously cited show good concordance between IFA and western blot results. It should be noted, however, that it is often necessary to absorb sera that give nonspecific staining with uninfected cells[68] before a correct result can be obtained. The nonspecific staining of nearly all sera can be removed by absorption except for a few that were found to contain antinuclear antibodies. Widespread use of the IFA has been impeded by the lack of FDA-licensed tests and the lack of standardization of in-house and commercial tests.

Radioimmunoprecipitation Assay

The radioimmunoprecipitation assay (RIPA) is another test that is sometimes performed as a supplemental test for EIA. Actively growing cells infected with HIV-1 or HIV-2 are exposed to a growth medium containing radioactive amino acids that become incorporated into the viral proteins.[46,69–72] Cell lysates prepared from these cells are first cleared of proteins that bind nonvirus-specific antibodies by absorbing them with a negative human control serum bound to protein A-Sepharose beads. The lysates are then mixed with the patient's serum and incubated until equilibrium is reached. The immune complexes are then absorbed with Protein A-Sepharose beads. Radioactive antibody–antigen complexes are eluted, and positive eluates are separated by sodium dodecyl sulfate–polyacrylamide gel electrophoresis (SDS-PAGE) to determine specific viral patterns. The binding patterns are similar to those of western blot.

This technique has the disadvantage of being very cumbersome and expensive and is, therefore, primarily a research tool. The advantages of RIPA is that it seems to be more sensitive than Western blot for antibodies to the *env* glycoproteins. Because RIPA uses a cell lysate rather than the lysate of pelleted virus, it contains the true envelope precursor (gp160) and external glycoprotein (gp120). Experience has shown that RIPA is very helpful in confirming HIV infection and in typing the infecting virus as HIV-1 or HIV-2.

Assaying for HIV Antibody in Dried Blood Specimens

For 30 years, state laboratories have screened newborns for metabolic disorders by testing blood specimens obtained by heel-sticks and collected on absorbent paper (Schleicher and Schuell No. 903, Keene, New Hampshire). Recently, it has been shown that antibodies to HIV can be detected in these newborn specimens and, because IgG antibodies are transferred to the fetus, the newborn blood specimens can be used to study the prevalence of HIV in women bearing liveborn infants.[73] More than 2 million infants have been tested by this method (unpublished data) in the CDC HIV Survey of Childbearing Women. A procedural manual describing all the laboratory techniques used in the Survey has been published.[74] Subsequent studies conducted by Genetic Systems (Seattle, Washington) and Organon Teknika (Durham, North Carolina) have shown that testing dried blood samples collected on S&S No. 903 filter paper from finger-sticks gives the same sensitivity and specificity as testing serum and plasma. Subsequent to these findings the FDA has licensed the EIAs produced by these companies for use with dried blood samples.

Testing dried blood spot samples requires that the antibodies be eluted overnight in sample diluent provided by the manufacturer of the EIA. A $\frac{1}{4}$-in. spot punched from the filter paper contains approximately 5.0 μl of serum. The dilution of the antibody in the eluate may be more concentrated than that used in the EIA test and will require further dilution (see kit insert) before testing. At this point the assay is performed in the same manner as a test with serum or plasma. As with other specimens, initially reactive specimens are retested in duplicate. If possible, new eluates should be prepared for the retest. However, the blinded nature of the Survey of Childbearing Women means that the repeat testing and the supplemental testing must be performed on the same eluate. Eluates have been found to be stable at 4°C for at least 1 week. Repeatedly reactive specimens are confirmed by testing with western blot. In the Survey of Childbearing Women, because limited quantities of sample were available, a special modification of western blot is used that permits testing of

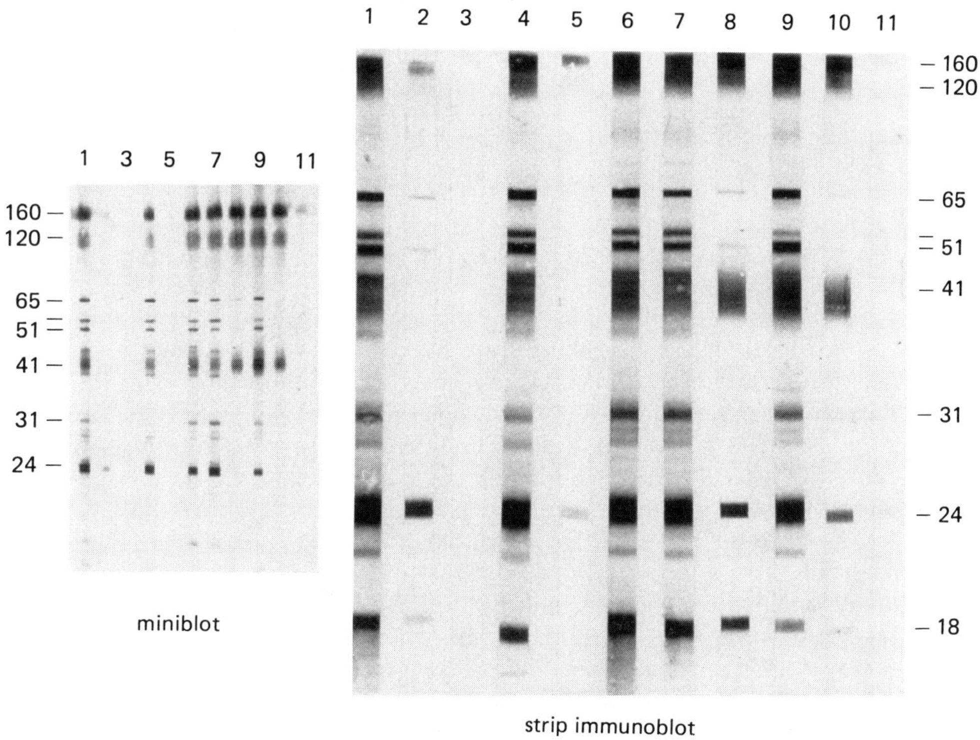

FIGURE 5.8. Comparison of "mini" western blot technique to FDA-licensed Du Pont/Biotech test. Same 11 sera were run in each test.

70 μl of a 1:100 dilution of antibody.[74] An example of this test as compared to the FDA licensed western blot is shown in Figure 5.8.

Collection of blood samples on absorbent paper has unique advantages for large-scale screening programs or for situations in which the collection, processing, and storage of serum or plasma specimens would be difficult or impossible. These samples can be collected by sticking the heel, finger, or ear, eliminating the need for venipuncture. Once collected and completely dried, the dried samples do not require refrigeration, and they can be mailed conveniently and inexpensively to a central laboratory for analysis. When protected from moisture, samples can be stored unrefrigerated for 30 days. For long-term storage, the samples should be placed in gas-impermeable bags with small packets of dessicant and stored at −20°C.

The disadvantages of testing dried blood samples are few but are important to note. Collection of appropriate samples is critical to accurate test results. The circles on the collection samples should be completely filled and saturated. Once collected the specimens must be thoroughly dried before being allowed to contact other surfaces or being placed in plastic bags. Detailed instuctions for collecting specimens have been published[74] and must be closely followed. Testing of samples must include the appropriate filter paper controls,[74] and testing laboratories should participate in a proficiency testing program that distributes specimens dried on filter paper. If all these recommendations are observed, results from testing dried blood spot samples will give the same results as obtained with serum or plasma.

Tests for HIV IgA and IgM Antibodies

Detection of infected infants born to seropositive mothers by serologic assays is difficult because HIV-reactive antibodies produced by the infant are obscured by large quantities of maternal immunoglobulin G (IgG). Passively acquired antibodies may persist for up to 18 months in the infant[75,76] with a mean of about 9 months. Consequently, only tests that can differentiate between antibodies of maternal and fetal origin are of diagnostic value. Assays that are specific for IgM or IgA seem best suited for this purpose because it is known that these antibodies do not cross the placenta.

Implementation of IgM and IgA assays has been hindered by the reported poor specificity of these tests.[77] It is generally agreed that the observed nonspecificity results from the incomplete removal and subsequent detection of maternal IgG. However, it has been shown that this problem can be eliminated by absorbing the antisera with an engineered recombinant form of streptococcal Protein G[78] (GammaBind™, Genex Corp., Gaithersberg, Maryland). Efficiency of removal of IgG was monitored by titration of IgG HIV antibody before and after absorption. In some cases three absorptions were required to completely remove IgG antibody.

Once the IgG antibodies have been removed, the IgA and IgG antibodies produced by the infant can be detected by an immunoblot procedure similar to that described in Figure 5.4. However, the IgA and IgM assays require that a class-specific antibody be used to prepare the conjugate. The assay for IgA HIV antibodies have been promising. Weiblen et al.[78] reported that they detected IgA antibodies in the sera of 66% of infected infants by the age of 6 months. On the other hand, IgM tests for HIV antibodies have been disappointing; only 33% of infected infants were positive for IgM antibodies at the same age. It is not clear whether the observed insensitivity is caused by the lack of early IgM antibody production or the poor sensitivity of the IgM assays. Conjugates for IgM antibodies are clearly inferior in sensitivity and background to IgA conjugates.

Sensitivity, Specificity, and Predictive Value of Serologic Tests

Is the test result positive or negative?—it would seem that this is a simple question with a simple answer. In fact, the answer is complex and requires that we understand several other concepts. First, we must introduce the concept of predictive value. Predictive value is defined by Galen and Gambino[79] as "how accurately a test predicts the presence or absence of disease." The answer to this question is based on the analysis of three variables: (1) *sensitivity*—the incidence of true-positive results in patients with disease; (2) *specificity*—the incidence of true-negative results in patients without disease; and (3) *prevalence*—the incidence (cases per 100,000) of the disease in the population being tested within a given time period.

The predictive value of a positive test (PPV) is defined as the percentage of positive results that are true-positives when the test is applied to a population containing both healthy and diseased subjects. The predictive value of a negative test (NPV) is the percentage of negative results that are true-negatives. As previously suggested this would depend on the number of false-positives and false-negatives produced by the test being used in relation to the number of true-positives and true-negatives and the prevalence of infection in the population. These relationships are illustrated in Table 5.4.

The ideal test would establish the presence or absence of infection in every individual screened. In other words, there would never be any false-positive or false-negative results. Unfortunately, there are no per-

TABLE 5.4. Predictive value of EIA tests for HIV antibody as applied to population containing both infected and uninfected subjects.

	Test results		
Disease state	Number of subjects with positive test results	Number of subjects with negative test results	Total
Number subjects with disease	TP[a]	FN	TP + FN
Number subjects without disease	FP	TN	FP + TN
Totals	TP + FP	FN + TN	TP + FP + FN + TN

[a] TP = true-positives, number of sick subjects correctly classified by test.
FP = false-positives, number of healthy subjects misclassified by test.
TN = true-negatives, number of healthy subjects correctly classified by test.
FN = false-negatives, number of sick subjects misclassified by test.

$$\text{Sensitivity (positivity in disease)} = \frac{TP}{TP + FN} \times 100$$

$$\text{Specificity (negativity in health)} = \frac{TN}{TN + FP} \times 100$$

$$\text{Predictive value of positive result} = \frac{TP}{TP + FP} \times 100$$

$$\text{Predictive value of negative result} = \frac{TN}{TN + FN} \times 100$$

fect tests. As large numbers of blood donors were screened, it became clear that the distribution of EIA test absorbance values did not assume a normal distribution but was positively skewed.[80] The cutoffs for each licensed test were set within the tail of this distribution such that 0.2–1.0% of random donors were initially reactive. Following FDA recommendations, these initially reactive samples were tested in duplicate. Units that were repeatedly reactive were discarded.

Licensed tests for HIV antibody are extremely sensitive (>99.8%) and specific (>99.8%). However, the prevalence of HIV infection in the populations being screened is low, usually less than 0.1%. The PPV of the EIA tests for screening blood donations (prevalence = 0.02%) using tests with sensitivity and specificity of 99.8% (Table 5.5) is low, 9.0%. This means that for every true-positive, nine other sera will be incorrectly identified as positive in the initial screening. As the prevalence of infection in the population increases, the incidence of false-positive results decreases (Figure 5.9). At a prevalence of 1.0%, the same EIA test will have a PPV of 83.4% (Table 5.6). If only the disposition of the blood was involved, EIA results might be sufficient. However, notification of donors testing positive was predicated on the ability to confirm the EIA reactivity.

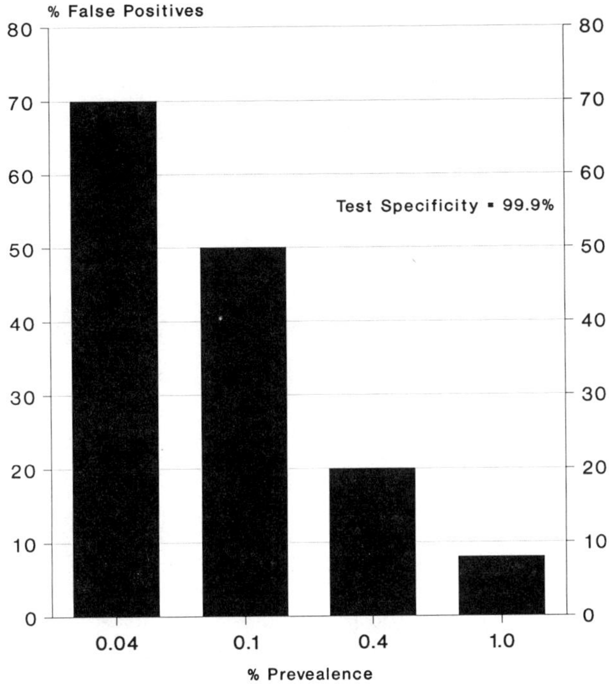

FIGURE 5.9. Percentage of false-positives decreases as prevalence of infection in population increases.

TABLE 5.5. Predictive value of EIA tests for HIV antibody as applied to population with prevalence of 0.02% infection.[a]

	Test results		
Disease state	Number of subjects with positive test results	Number of subjects with negative test results	Total
Subjects with disease	199	1	200
Subjects without disease	2000	997,800	999,800
Totals	2199	997,801	1,000,000

$$\text{Predictive value of a positive result} = \frac{199}{199 + 2000} \times 100 = 9.0\%$$

$$\text{Predictive value of a negative result} = \frac{997{,}800}{1 + 997{,}801} \times 100 = 100\%$$

[a] Assay sensitivity, 99.8%; assay specificity, 99.8%.

TABLE 5.6. Predictive value of EIA tests for HIV antibody as applied to population with prevalence of 1.0% infection.[a]

Disease state	Test results: Number of subjects with positive test results	Test results: Number of subjects with negative test results	Total
Subjects with disease	9980	20	10,000
Subjects without disease	1980	998,020	990,000
Totals	11,960	998,040	1,000,000

$$\text{Predictive value of a positive result} = \frac{9980}{9980 + 1980} \times 100 = 83.4\%$$

$$\text{Predictive value of a negative result} = \frac{998{,}020}{998{,}020 + 20} \times 100 = 100\%$$

[a] Assay sensitivity, 99.8%; assay specificity, 99.8%.

The problem of low PPV is addressed by the serial testing of the initially reactive subjects by additional EIAs and supplemental tests such as western blot. Therefore, the PPV of the individual tests become less important in relationship to the probability of a false-positive test (P_{FP}), the probability of a false-negative test (P_{FN}) and the PPV of the recommended HIV testing algorithm. In our example, let S^+ stand for a positive subject and S^- stand for a negative; let E^+ be a positive EIA test result and E^- be a negative EIA test result; W^+ and W^- are the same for western blot results. Then the prevalence is the probability that the subject is positive: $P(S^+) = 0.001$ (0.1%). The sensitivity of the EIA is $P(E^+/S^+) = 0.998$, and the specificity is $P(E^-/S^-) = 0.998$. For the western blot $P(W^+/S^+) = 0.996$ and $P(W^-/S^-) = 0.996$. The formula for the P_{FP} and P_{FN} for one test is as follows:

$$P_{FP} = \frac{P(T/S^-)[1 - P(S^+)]}{P(T/S^-) + P(S^+)[P(T/S^+) - P(T/S^-)]}$$

We need the $P(T/S^+)$ and $P(T/S^-)$ for our entire four-test algorithm to substitute in the formula.

The $P(T/S^+)$ is the probability that the algorithm gives a positive result given that the subject is a true-positive. The possible outcomes of the tests that will lead to a positive conclusion are ++++ OR +−++ OR ++−+. Assuming that the tests are independent, given that the subject is positive, we have:

$$\begin{aligned} P(T/S^+) &= P_{T+} \\ &= P(++++ \text{ OR } +-++ \text{ OR } ++-+) \\ &= 0.998 \times 0.998 \times 0.998 \times 0.996 + 2 \times 0.998 \times 0.998 \\ &\quad \times (1 - 0.998) \times 0.996 \\ &= 0.9940040239, \end{aligned}$$

and if the subject is negative:

$$P(T/S^-) = (1 - 0.998)^3 \times (1 - 0.996) + 2 \times (1 - 0.998)^2 \times 0.998 \times (1 - 0.996) = 0.000000031968$$

Substituting in the above expressions, we get:

$$P_{FP} = 0.00003212761425452, \text{ or 32 per 1 million tests.}$$

The PPV = 0.999967679 or essentially 100%.

The probability of a false-negative tests is P_{FN} = 0.000007987 or 8 per million tests. The NPV is essentially 100%.

HIV Antigen Detection

Assay Methods

The first use of HIV antigen detection was for minitoring viral antigen in cell culture supernatants, thereby providing direct confirmation of reverse transcriptase assay results.[81] In 1986, commercial EIA tests for HIV core antigen (p24) became available (Abbott Laboratories, E.I. du Pont de Nemours) for detecting viral antigen in serum, plasma, and cerebrospinal fluid. In 1988, the Abbott Laboratories HIV antigen EIA was licensed by the FDA for diagnostic testing. Several other companies offer tests for investigational use. The principle of detection for HIV antigen tests involves incubating the patient's specimen with anti-HIV-1 capture antibody bound to a solid support, such as polystyrene beads of microplate wells. After washing, the immune complex bound to the solid support is incubated with a second anti-HIV-1 antibody to form a sandwich. This second antibody, in some assays, is conjugated to an enzyme that subsequently is reacted with substrate. The resulting color change can be detected by the increase in absorbance at a specific wavelength, which provides a quantitative measurement of the amount of HIV antigen present in the test sample.

Other assays (Figure 5.10) use an unlabeled second antibody (rabbit anti-HIV-1) followed by enzyme-conjugated goat anti-rabbit IgG. After the final wash the amount of HIV antigen present in the immune complex is detected as before by the color change resulting from the enzyme conversion of substrate. The second assay described is said to be more sensitive than the first because of the amplification provided by the addition of the second antibody. Both types of assays quantitate the amount of unbound HIV antigen present in the patient's sample by comparison to a standard curve prepared from dilutions of known amounts of HIV antigen. The detectable limit of these assays has been reported to be between 10 and 30 pg/ml.[82–85]

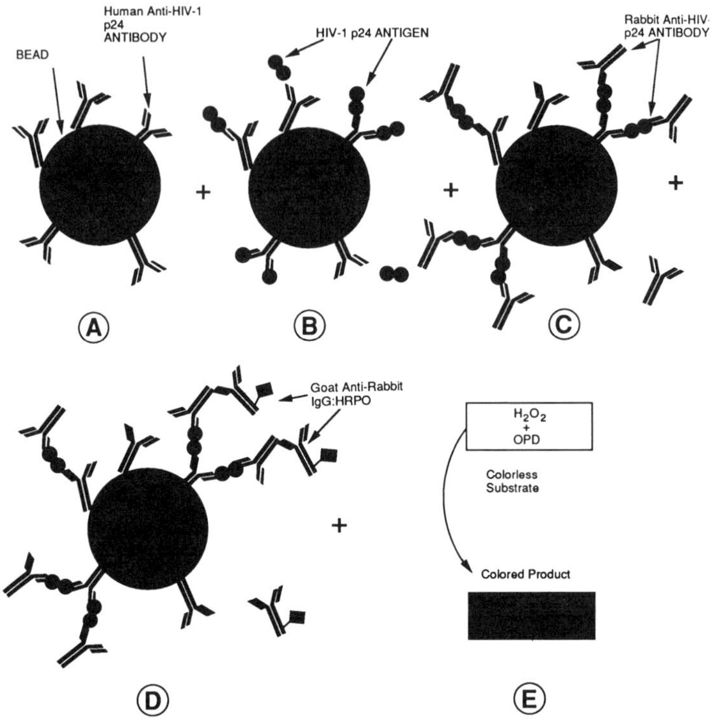

FIGURE 5.10. Configuration for p24 antigen test.

All reactive specimens should be confirmed by a specific neutralization assay to verify the presence of HIV-1 antigen. Neutralization involves preincubating the specimen with human anti-HIV antibody before performing the HIV-1 antigen EIA. If antigen is present, the neutralizing antibody will form an immune complex that prevents binding of the HIV-1 antigen to the HIV-1 antibody bound to the solid support. Reactive specimens are considered confirmed when neutralization results in a reduction of absorbance by at least 50% when compared with the specimen in which human serum nonreactive with HIV-1 is used in place of neutralizing antibody.

Applications of Antigen Testing

Considerable effort has been expended to demonstrate that antigen testing should be added to the battery of tests used to screen blood used for transfusion. Insertion of the HIV antigen test was proposed to close or shorten the window period (see Figure 5.1) between infection and seroconversion. The usefulness of the HIV antigen test in this application will depend on the prevalence of the infection in the population being tested and the length of the window period. In low-prevalence populations, such as blood donors, the routine use of antigen screening does not appear to be justified. Results from three separate studies testing several hundred thousand blood donors showed that antigen detection was no more sensitive than routine antibody screening for detecting HIV-infected donors.[86,87] For high-risk asymptomatic populations, the HIV antigen EIA may prove increasingly useful in diagnostic and prognostic applications. HIV antigen has been detected in early infection of seronegative individuals who are members of a high-risk group or who present with the acute HIV infection syndrome before seroconversion.[88–91] However, most HIV-infected individuals become HIV antigen negative shortly after seroconversion.[91]

Antigen testing has also been shown to be a useful tool in several clinical situations. There is a correlation between the onset of antigenemia and the progression to disease. Antigen testing is also useful in determining HIV infection in neonates born to HIV-infected mothers. And, finally HIV antigen testing can be an effective tool for assessing the therapeutic efficacy of different antiviral drugs. Unfortunately, the low prevalence of antigenemia observed in asymptomatic, HIV-infected populations may limit its usefulness to drug studies involving symptomatic patients in whom the prevalence of antigenemia is much higher. It has been shown that the sensitivity of the test increases with clinical progression of disease, showing 4% positivity in asymptomatic patients, 56% with patients having AIDS-related diseases, and 70% in AIDS patients.[92]

Antigen testing has several recognized limitations. Testing of hemolyzed or lipemic specimens should be avoided. If specimens must be stored, they may be refrigerated at 4°C for 1 week or frozen. Multiple freeze-thaw cycles of frozen samples should be avoided. Furthermore, it is important to emphasize that these tests appear to detect only free p24 antigen. In patients who have a high titer of p24 antibody, p24 antigen appears to be complexed with antibody and is difficult to detect.[92] This is further supported by the observation that persons who are p24 antigen positive after exposure become negative when they seroconvert.[93] Patients again become antigen positive as their p24 antibody falls during progression to the symptomatic state.[91,94]

At the present time, HIV antigen EIA provides a valuable additional tool to antibody testing for the detection of HIV infection. Positive results on the antigen EIA, confirmed by the neutralization test, provide direct evidence of the presence of the virus. However recently developed tests (e.g., PCR) that detect HIV RNA or DNA have surpassed the antigen EIA in sensitivity and specificity. However, antigen testing still has value in situations in which molecular techniques such as PCR are not available.

Conclusions

Sensitive, specific, and inexpensive tests for HIV antibodies have permitted the implementation of effective screening programs to protect the blood supply and to conduct seroprevalence studies to measure the spread of the disease. It has also permitted accurate diagnosis of HIV infection in asymptomatic carriers. These programs have dramatically reduced the rate of spread of the disease in the United States and many other parts of the world. As the AIDS epidemic continues to spread, there will be sustained need for more sensitive and quantitative assays. Tests of higher sensitivity will be needed to permit earlier diagnosis of infection, which will become increasingly important as effective therapeutic interventions are developed to prevent the disease. Tests having greater sensitivity will be needed to reduce the number of false-positives that result from mass screening of low-prevalence populations. Tests should be developed that will detect infection in neonates immediately after birth to allow intervention therapies.

Direct tests that measure viral antigens or the viral genome have progressed rapidly. These tests have progressed from experimental procedures that required several days to perform and cost several hundred dollars to methods that can be completed in a single day. These tests will continue to improve and will assume an important role in HIV testing. However, in the immediate future antibody testing will retain the dominant position in disease control. Considerable progress can be expected in the development of more rapid, sensitive, and specific serologic tests.

Acknowledgment. Statistical calculations performed by Robert H. Byers, Jr., Ph.D., Chief, Statistical Section DHA, CDC.

References

1. Centers for Disease Control. Provisional public health service inter-agency recommendations for screening donated blood and plasma for antibody to the virus causing acquired immunodeficiency syndrome. MMWR 1985;34:1–5.
2. Centers for Disease Control. Public Health Service guidelines for counseling and antibody testing to prevent HIV infection and AIDS. MMWR 1987;36:509–515.
3. Centers for Disease Control. Update: serologic testing for antibody to human immunodeficiency virus. MMWR 1988;39:833–840.
4. Martin PW, Burger DR, Caouette S, Goldstein AS, Peetoom F. Importance of confirmatory tests after strongly positive HTLV-III screening tests. N Engl J Med 1986;317:1577–1578.
5. Centers for Disease Control. AIDS due to HIV-2 infection—New Jersey. MMWR 1988;37:33–35.
6. Centers for Disease Control. 1987–1989. Surveillance for HIV-2 infections in blood donors—United States. MMWR 1988;39:829–831.

7. O'Brien TR, Schable CA, Polon C, Stewart A, VanDevanter N, Schochetman G, et al. HIV-2 infections in the United States [abstract]. In: VIth International Conference on AIDS, Vol. 2:245.
8. George JR, Rayfield MA Phillips S, Heyward WL, Krebs JW, Odehouri K, et al. Efficacies of U.S. Food and Drug Administration—licensed HIV-1 screening enzyme immunoassays for detecting antibodies to HIV-2. 1990; AIDS 4:321–326.
9. Schumacher RT, Howard J, Ayres L, Pista A, Avillez F, Garrett P. Cross-reactivity of anti-HIV-2 positive serum in US FDA licensed screening tests for anti-HIV-1 [abstract]. In: VIth International Conference on AIDS, Vol. 3:245.
10. Smith TF, Srinivasan A, Schochetman G, Marcus M, Myers G. The phylogenetic history of immunodeficiency viruses. Nature (London) 1988;333:573.
11. Dierksheide WC. Medical decisions: interpreting clinical tests. ASM News 1987;53:677.
12. Centers for Disease Control. Update: acquired immunodeficiency syndrome—United States. MMWR 1987;36:522–526.
13. Reesink HW, Lelie PN, Huisman JG, Schasberg M, Gonsalves C, Aaij C, et al. Evaluation of six enzyme immunoassays for antibody against human immunodeficiency virus. Lancet 1986;ii:483–486.
14. Schochetman G, Epstein JS, Zuck TF. Serodiagnosis of infection with the AIDS virus and other human retroviruses. Annu Rev Microbiol 1989;43: 629–659.
15. Cooper DA, Gold J, Maclean P, Donovan R, Finlayson R, Barnes TG, et al. Acute AIDS retrovirus infection: definition of a clinical illness associated with seroconversion. Lancet 1985;i:537–540.
16. Esteban JI, Shih JW, Tai CC, Bodner AJ, Kay JWD, Alter HJ. Importance of western blot analysis in predicting infectivity of anti-HTLV-III/LAV positive blood. Lancet 1985;ii:1083–1086.
17. Gaines H, Von Sydow M, Sonnerborg A, Albert J, Czajkowski J, Pehrson PO, et al. Antibody response in primary human immunodeficiency virus infection. Lancet 1987;i:1249–1253.
18. Ho DD, Sarngadharan MG, Resnick L, Dimarzo-Veronese F, Rota TR, Hirsch MS. Primary human T-lymphotropic virus type III infection. Ann Intern Med 1985;103:880–883.
19. Kumar P, Pearson JE, Martin DH, Leech SH, Buisseret PD, Bezbak HC, et al. Transmission of human immunodeficiency virus by transplantation of a renal allograft, with development of the acquired immunodeficiency syndrome. Ann Intern Med 1987;106:244–245.
20. Marlink RG, Allan JS, McLane MF, Essex M, Anderson KC, Groopman JE. Low sensitivity of ELISA testing in early HIV infection. N Engl J Med 1986;315:1549.
21. Ulstrup JC, Skaug K, Figenschau KJ, Orstavik I, Brunn JN, Petersen G. Sensitivity of Western blotting (compared with ELISA and immunofluorescence) during seroconversion after HTLV-III infection. Lancet 1986;i: 1151–1152.
22. Anderson KC, Gorgone BC, Marlink RC, Ferriani R, Essex ME, Benz PM, et al. Transfusion-acquired human immunodeficiency virus infection among immunocompromised persons. Ann Intern Med 1986;105:519–527.

23. Bedarida G, Cambie G, D'Agostino F, D'Agostino F, Ronsivalle JB. HIV IgM antibodies in risk groups who are seronegative on ELISA testing. Lancet 1986;ii:570–571.
24. Parry JV, Mortimer PP. Place of IgM antibody testing in HIV serology. Lancet 1986;ii:979–980.
25. Bedarida G, Cambie G, D'Agostino F, Ronsivalle E, Berto E, Grisi ME, et al. Anti-IgM screening for HIV. Lancet 1986;ii:1456.
26. Ward JW, Grindon AJ, Feorino PM, Schable C, Parvin M, Allen JR. Laboratory and epidemiologic evaluation of an enzyme immunoassay for antibodies to HTLV-III. JAMA 1986;256:357–361.
27. Blanton M, Balakrishnan K, Dumaswala U, Zelenski K, Greenwalt TJ. HLA antibodies in blood donors with reactive screening tests for antibody to the immunodeficiency virus. Transfusion (Philadelphia) 1987;27:118–119.
28. Kuhnl P, Seidl S, Holzberger G. HLA DR4 antibodies cause positive HTLV-III antibody ELISA results. Lancet 1985;i:1222–1223.
29. Smith DM, Dewhurst S, Shepherd S, Volsky DJ, Goldsmith JC. False-positive enzyme-linked immunosorbent assay reactions for antibody to human immunodeficiency virus in a population of midwestern patients with congenital bleeding disorders. Transfusion (Philadelphia) 1987;27:112.
30. Mendenhall CL, Roselle GA, Grossman CJ, Rouster SD, Weesner RE, Dumaswala U. False positive tests for HTLV-III antibodies in alcoholic patients with hepatitis. N Engl J Med 1986;314:921–922.
31. Peterman TA, Lang GR, Mikos NJ, et al. HTLV-III/LAV infection in hemodialysis patients. JAMA 1986;255:2324–2326.
32. Fleming DW, Cochi SL, Steece RS, Hull HF. Acquired immunodeficiency syndrome in low-incidence areas. JAMA 1987;258:785–787.
33. World Health Organization. Operational characteristics of commercially available assays to determine antibodies to HIV-1. Global Program for AIDS/Biomedical Research Unit 1989;89.4.
34. Crofts JN, Maskill WJ, Healey DS, Gust ID. Particle agglutination test for anti-HIV. Lancet 1987;ii:797–798.
35. Yoshida T, Matsui T, Kobayashi S, Yamamoto N. Evaluation of passive particle agglutination test for antibody to human immunodeficiency virus. J Clin Microbiol 1987;25:1433–1437.
36. Riggens CH, Thorn RM. Visually read HIV immunoassays. Lancet 1989; i:671–672.
37. Spielberg F, Ryder RW, Harris J, Heyward WL, Kabeya CL, Kifuani NF, et al. Field testing and comparative evaluation of rapid, visually read screening assays for antibody to human immunodeficiency virus. Lancet 1989; i:580–584.
38. World Health Organization. Operational characteristics of commercially available assays to determine antibodies to HIV-1 and/or HIV-2 in human sera. Report 2. Global Program for AIDS/Biomedical Research Unit 1990; 90.1.
39. DeCock KM, Maran M, Kouadio JC, Porter A, LaFontaine MF, Gnore E, et al. Rapid test for distinguishing HIV-1 and HIV-2. Lancet 1990;336:757.
40. Tsang VCW, Peralta JM, Simons AR. Enzyme-linked immunoelectrotransfer blot techniques (EITB) for studying the specificities of antigens and antibodies separated by gel electrophoresis. Methods Enyzmol 1983;92:377–391.

41. Esteban JI, Shih JW, Tai CC, Bodner AJ, Kay JWD, Alter HJ. Importance of Western blot analysis in predicting infectivity of anti-HTLV-III/LAV positive blood. Lancet 1985;ii:1083–1086.
42. Goudsmit J, Lange JMA, Paul DA, Dawson GJ, Antigenemia and antibody titers to core and envelope antigens in AIDS, ARC ad subclinical HIV infection. J. Infect Dis 1987;155:558–560.
43. Lange J, Coutinho RA, Krone WJA, Verdonch LF, Danner SA, Van Der Noordaa J, et al. Distinct IgG recognitional patterns during progression of subclinical and clinical infection with lymphadenopathy associated virus/human T lymphotropic virus. Br Med J 1986;292:228–230.
44. Lange, J, Paul DA, Huisman HG, DeWolf F, Van Den Berg J, Van Der Noordaa J, et al. Persistent HIV antigenemia and decline of HIV core antibodies associated with transition to AIDS. Br Med J 1986;293:1459–1462.
45. McDougal JS, Kennedy MS, Nicholson JKA, Spira TJ, Jaffe HW, Kaplan JE, et al. Antibody response to human immuno-deficiency virus in homosexual men: relation of antibody specificity, titer, and isotype to clinical status, severity of immunodeficiency, and disease progression. J Clin Invest 1987;80:316–324.
46. Barin F, McLane MF, Allan JS, Lee TH. Virus envelope protein of HTLV-III represents major target antigen for antibodies in AIDS patients. Science 1985;118:1094–1096.
47. Essex M, Allan J, Kanki P, McLane MF, Malone G, Kitchen L, et al. Antigens of human T-lymphotropic virus type III/lymphadenopathy-associated virus. Ann Intern Med 1985;103:700–703.
48. Kitchen LW, Barin F, Sullivan JL, McLane MF, Brettler DB, Levine PH, et al. Aeitology of AIDS-antibodies to human T-cell leukemia virus (type III) in hemophiliacs. Nature (London) 1984;312:367–369.
49. Pinter A, Honnen WJ, Tilley SA, Bona C, Zaghonani H, Gorney MK, et al. Oligomeric structure of gp41, the transmembrane protein of human immunodeficiency virus type 1. J Virol 1989;63:2674–2679.
50. Zolla-Pazner S, Gorny MK, Honnen WJ, Pinter A. Reinterpretation of human immunodeficiency virus western blot patterns. N Engl J Med 1989; 320:1280–1281.
51. DeCock KM, Porter A, Kouadio J, Maran M, Gnaore E, Adjorlolo G, et al. Rapid and specific diagnosis of HIV-1 and HIV-2 infections: an evaluation of testing strategies. AIDS 1990;4:875–878.
52. Centers for Disease Control. Interpretation and use of the western blot assay for serodiagnosis of human immunodeficiency virus type 1 infections. MMWR 1989;38(S-7):1–7.
53. Weber JN, Clapham P-R, Neiss RA, Parker D, Roberts C, Duncan J, et al. Human immunodeficiency virus infection in 2 cohorts of homosexual men—neutralizing sera and association of anti-gag antibody with prognosis. Lancet 1987;i:119–222.
54. World Health Organization. Proposed criteria for interpreting results from the Western blot assays for HIV-1, HIV-2, and HTLV-1/HTLV-II. WHO Wkly Epidemiol Rec 1990;37:281–283.
55. Burke DS, Brundage JF, Herbold JR, Berner W, Gardner LI, Gunzenhauser JD, et al. Human immunodeficiency virus infections among civilian applicants

for United States military service, October 1985 to March 1986. N Engl J Med 1987;317:131–136.
56. Kleinman S, Fitzpatrick L, Secord K. Follow-up testing and notification of anti-HIV western blot atypical (indeterminant) donors. Transfusion (Philadelphia) 1988;28:280–282.
57. Dock NL, Lamberson HV, O'Brien TA, Tribe DE, Alexander SS, and Poiesz BJ. Evaluation of atypical human immunodeficiency virus immunoblot reactivity in blood donors. Transfusion (Philadelphia) 1988;28:412–418.
58. Josephson SC, Swack NS, Ramirez MT, Hausler WJ. Investigation of atypical western blot (immunoblot) reactivity involving core proteins of human immunodeficiency virus type 1. J Clin Microbiol 1989;37:922–927.
59. Jackson JB, MacDonald KL, Cadwell J, Sullivan C, Kline WE, Hanson M, et al. Absence of HIV infection in blood donors with indeterminate Western blot tests for antibody to HIV-1. N Engl J Med 1990;322:217–222.
60. Dock NL, Kleinman SH, Rayfield MA, Schable CA, Williams AE, Dodd RY. Status of human immunodeficiency virus infection in individuals with persistently indeterminate western blot patterns: prospective studies in a low prevalence population. Arch Intern Med 1991;151:525–530.
61. Cable RG, Kakaiya RM, Roberts SC, Martin CR. Follow-up testing of blood donors found to be enzyme immunoassay positive/western blot negative for HTLV-III antibody. JAMA 1986;256:40–41.
62. Blumberg RS, Sandstrom EG, Paradis TJ, Nuemeyer DN, Sarngadharan MG, Hartshorn KL, et al. Detection of human T-cell lymphotropic virus type III-related antigens and anti-human T-cell lymphotropic virus type III antibodies by anticomplementary immunofluorescence. J Clin Microbiol 1986; 23:1072–1077.
63. Gallo D, Diggs JL, Shell GR, Dailey PJ, Hoffman MN, Riggs JL. Comparison of detection of antibody to the acquired immune deficiency syndrome virus by enzyme immunoassay, immunofluorescence and Western blot methods. J Clin Microbiol 1986;23:1049–1051.
64. Kaminsky LS, McHugh T, Stites D, Volberding P, Henle W, Levy JA. High prevalence of antibodies to acquired immune deficiency syndrome (AIDS)-associated retrovirus (ARV) in AIDS and related conditions but not in order disease states. Proc Natl Acad Sci USA 1985;82:5535–5539.
65. Levy JA, Hoffman AD, Kramer SM, Landis JM, Shimbukuro JM, Oshiro LS. Isolation of lymphocytopathic retroviruses from San Francisco patients with AIDS. Science 1984;225:840–842.
66. Pan LZ, Cheng-Mayer C, Levy JA. Patterns of antibody response in individuals infected with the human immuno-deficiency virus. J Infect Dis 1987;155: 626–632.
67. Popovic M, Sarngadharan MG, Read E, Gallo RC. Detection, isolation, and continuous production of cytopathic retroviruses (HTLV-III) from patients with AIDS and pre-AIDS. Science 1984;224:497–500.
68. Gallo D, Diggs JL, Shell GR, Dailey MN, Hoffman MN, Riggs JL. Comparison of detection of antibody to the acquired immune deficiency syndrome virus by enzyme immunoassay, immunofluorescence, and western blot methods. J Clin Microbiol 1986;23:1049–1051.
69. Allan JS, Coligan JE, Lee TH, Sodroski JG, Lee TH. Immunogenic nature of a pol gene product of HTLV-III/LAV. Blood 1987;69:331–333.

70. Barre-Sinoussi F, Mathur-Wagh U, Rey F, Brun-Vezinet F, Yancovitz SR, Rouzioux C, et al. Isolation of lymphadenopathy-associated virus (LAV) and detection of LAV antibodies from US patients with AIDS. JAMA 1985;253: 1737–1739.
71. Kanki PJ, Barin F, M'Boup S, Allan JS, Pomet-Lemonne JO, Marlink R, et al. New human T-lymphotropic retrovirus to simian T-lymphotropic virus type III $(STLV\text{-}III)_{AGM}$. Science 1986;232:238–243.
72. Schupbach J, Popovic M, Gilden RV, Gonda MA, Sargadharan MG, Galla RC. Serological analysis of a subgroup of human T-lymphotropic retroviruses (HTLV-III) associated with AIDS. Science 1984;224:503–505.
73. Hoff R, Berardi V, Weiblen BJ, Mahoney-Trout L, Mitchell ML, Grady GF. Seroprevalence of human immuno-deficiency virus among childbearing women. N Engl J Med 1988;318:525–530.
74. George JR, Hannon WH, Jones W, Kent PT, Hoff R, Weiblen BJ, et al. Serologic assays for human immunodeficiency virus antibody in dried-blood specimens collected on filter paper from neonates. U.S. Dept. of Health and Human Services, Public Health Service, Centers for Disease Control and National Institute of Child Health and Human Development, NIH, Bethesda MD:1989.
75. The European Collaborative Study. Mother-to-child transmission of HIV infection. Lancet 1988;i:1039–1042.
76. Mok JQ, Giaquinto, C, DeRossi A, Grosch-Worner I, Ades AE, Peckham CS. Infants born to mothers sero-positive for human immunodeficiency virus. Lancet 1987;i:1164–1167.
77. Jendis JB, Tomasik Z, Hunziker U, Nada D, Seger R, Wetzel JC, et al. Evaluation of diagnostic tests for HIV infection in infants born to HIV-infected mothers in Switzerland. AIDS 1988;2:273–279.
78. Weiblen BJ, Lee FK, Cooper ER, Landesman SH, McIntosh K, Harris JS, Early diagnosis of HIV infection in infants by detection of IgA HIV antibodies. Lancet 1990;335:988–990.
79. Galen RS, Gambino SR. Beyond Normality: The Predictive Value and Efficiency of Medical Diagnosis. New York: Wiley, 1975.
80. Britz JA, Rolon N, Hill T, Page E, Geltosky J. Interpreting HIV ELISA reactivity: alternatives to western blot. J Clin Lab Anal 1988;2:174–181.
81. Feorino P, Forrester B, Schable C, Warfield D, Schochetman G. Comparison of antigen assay and reverse transcriptase assay for detecting human immunodeficiency virus in culture. J Clin Microbiol 1987;25:2344–2346.
82. Goudsmit J, DeWolf F, Paul DA, Epstein LG, Lange JMA, Krone JA, et al. Expression of human immunodeficiency virus antigen (HIV-Ag) in serum and cerebrospinal fluid during acute and chronic infection. Lancet 1986,ii:177–180.
83. Goudsmit J, Lange JMA, Paul Da, Dawson GJ. Antigenemia and antibody titers to core and envelope antigens in AIDS, AIDS-related complex, and subclinical human immunodeficiency virus infection. J Infect Dis 1987;155: 558–560.
84. Barr PJ, Stimer KS, Sabin EA, Parkes D, George-Nasciment C, Stephans JC, et al. Antigenicity and immunogenicity of domains of the human immunodeficiency virus (HIV) envelope polypeptide expressed in the yeast *Saccharomyces cerevisiae*. Vaccine 1987;5(2):90–101.

85. Barr PJ, Power MD, Lee-Ng CT, Gibson HL, Luciw A, Expression of active human immunodeficiency virus reverse transcriptase in *Saccharomyces cerevisiae*. Bio Technol 1987;5:86–89.
86. Alter H, Epstein JS, Swenson SG, Menitove JE, Ward JW, Kaslow RA, et al. Collaborative study to evaluate HIV Ag (HIV-Ag) screening for blood donors. Transfusion (Philadelphia) 1989;29 (Suppl 7s):56 (abstr 5202).
87. Backer U, Weinauer F, Gathof AG, Eberle J. HIV antigen screening in blood donors. In: Abstracts, IVth International Conference on AIDS, Vol. 2. International AIDS Committee, 1988:364.
88. Gaines H, Albert J, Von Sydow M, Sonnerborg A, Chiodi F, Ehrnst A, et al. HIV antigenaemia and virus isolation from plasma during primary HIV infection. Lancet 1987;i:1317–1318.
89. Kessler H, Blaauw B, Spear J, Paul DA, Falk LA, Landay A. Diagnosis of human immunodeficiency virus infection in seronegative homosexuals presenting with an acute viral syndrome. JAMA 1987;258:1196–1199.
90. Wall R, Denning D, Amos A. HIV antigenaemia in acute HIV infection. Lancet 1987;i:566.
91. Von Sydow M, Gaines H, Sonnerborg A, Forsgren M, Pehrson PO, Strannegard O. Antigen detection in primary HIV infection. Br Med J 1988;295: 238–240.
92. Kenny C, Parkin J, Undershill G, Shah N, Burnell B, Osborne E, Jeffries DJ. HIV antigen testing. Lancet 1987;i:565–566.
93. Lange J, Goudsmit J. Decline of antibody reactivity to HIV core protein secondary to increased production of HIV antigen. Lancet 1987;i:448.
94. Allain J, Laurian Y, Paul DA, Senn D. Serological markers in early stages of human immunodeficiency virus infection in homophiliacs. Lancet 1986;ii: 1233–1236.

6
Quality Control for Serologic Testing

J. RICHARD GEORGE

The development and subsequent licensure by the U.S. Food and Drug Administration (FDA) of enzyme immunoassays (EIA) for human immunodeficrency virus (HIV) antibody provided a low-cost test that was well suited for diagnosis, mass screening of populations, and testing blood donations for HIV infection. Each year the number of tests performed as well as the number of laboratories performing tests increases in the United States, but programs for quality control (QC) of laboratory testing have not kept pace. Standard panels of serum for quality control and evaluation of EIA and western blot tests are not generally available. Quality control programs for serologic tests are crude compared to the sophisticated computer-driven programs used in clinical chemistry laboratories. In fact, some serology laboratories do no more than run the controls supplied by the kit manufacturer. Some serology laboratories, however, have adapted the QC procedures similar in design to those used for clinical chemistry to monitor testing for HIV infections. This chapter will describe these adaptations and recommend a simple and inexpensive system for quality control of HIV tests.

Quality assurance is the dynamic and ongoing process of monitoring the testing system for reproducibility that permits corrective action when established criteria are not met. Those techniques include statistical quality control procedures as well as procedures for method selection, method evaluation, preventive maintenance, in-service training, and laboratory management. Quality control is the study of those errors which are the responsibility of the laboratory and of the procedures used to recognize and minimize them. This study includes all errors arising within the laboratory between the receipt of the specimen and the dispatch of the test results report. On some occasions, the responsibility of the laboratory may extend to the collection of the appropriate specimen, method and time of collection, and the type of collection tube used.

Quality control requires the involvement of each technician and supervisor working in the laboratory. Quality control relies on the technicians to identify and to solve problems. Therefore, supervisors and employees must work closely together. Every employee should have an understanding of the quality control system. Everyone should be working to achieve zero error. There is *no minimum average acceptable* quality. Do it right the first time. Do not make mistakes. *Quality is free if produced the first time.*[1]

Preparation of Quality Control Materials

One of the objectives of quality control is to ensure that the results obtained in an EIA or western blot test performed today gives results that are qualitatively and quantitatively the same as those produced last week or last year. Further, that result must accurately reflect the infection status of the patient. This must be true even if the laboratory has changed testing methods during that time. An essential component required for that assurance is a pool of quality control materials for which a continuum of results is available. For HIV serology, the control material required would be pools of positive and negative sera for use in the testing algorithms. These pools should be large enough that they last for 6 to 12 months before new serum pools must be prepared.

Most laboratories find it difficult to obtain a single serum in sufficient quantity to last the required time. Therefore, the easier solution is to prepare pools of serum from unused samples sent in for analysis. In some ways these pools may be superior to a single donor because they represent individuals in different stages of infection (asymptomatic to AIDS patients), and these donors may represent different types of EIA and western blot reactivities. Preparation of serum pools has been well described[2] and begins by selecting only clear, straw-colored serum specimens. Plasma specimens should not be mixed with serum as they will clot even after recalcification. Turbid, chylous, hemolyzed, or icteric serum should not be used.

First, a pool of sera that is negative for HIV-1 antibody by EIA is prepared. This pool will be used as a diluent for the HIV-1 antibody-positive pool as well as for the negative control for EIA and western blot. All specimens are pooled; 0.01% sodium ethylmercurithiosalicylic acid is added, and the pool is mixed on a stirrer at 4°C overnight to assure homogeneity. The serum pool is filtered through a 10-μm-pore-size glass prefilter and then a 0.22-μm-pore-size sterile membrane filter. The final pool is tested by western blot and must not produce any bands on HIV-1 and HIV-2 strips.

The HIV-1 antibody-positive pool is prepared by pooling sera found to be positive by EIA and western blot. The pool of sera is filtered as was described. Dilutions of the positive pool from 1:2 to 1:2048 are prepared in the antibody-negative diluent. Each dilution of the pool should be tested in quadruplicate by EIA test and plotted as shown in Figure 6.1.

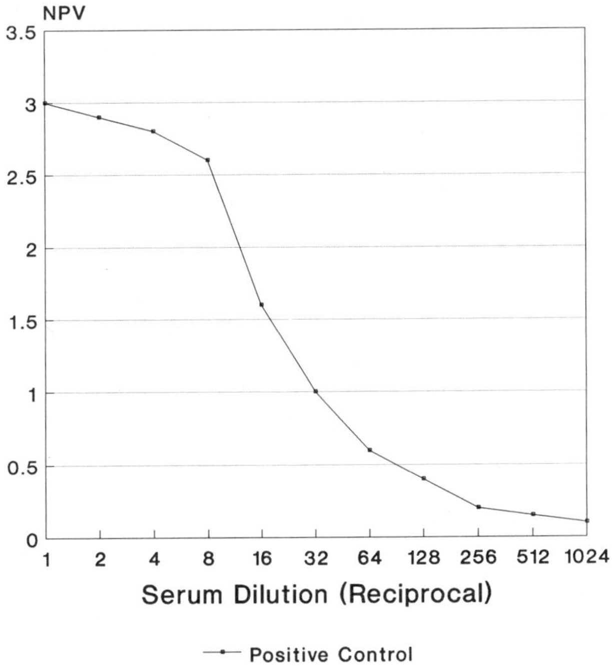

FIGURE 6.1. Titration of HIV-positive serum pool by enzyme immunoassay. Curve shows positive control.

The dilutions found to be on the "straight-line" part of the curve (1:8 to 1:128) are then tested by western blot. This analysis is used to select the dilution factor for the control pool. An appropriate positive control should have an absorbance close to the cutoff but sufficiently above it so that it will not often test negative because of the normal variability of the test. Frequent out-of-control signals when the assay is operating correctly will be ignored. The positive control pool should have (1) a sample/cutoff ratio of approximately 3 [this recommendation might need to be modified for assays in which the cutoff values tend to be high (>0.5)], and (2) should give clear, distinct bands for the HIV-1 structural proteins (gp160/120, p65, p55, p51, gp41, p32, p24, p17) on western blot.

Once prepared, the positive and negative control sera should be dispensed into quantities sufficient for 1 week of testing when controls are run in each assay microplate. Aliquots should be stored at −20°C or lower. Once thawed, the controls are used for 1 week and then discarded. In-house controls should be placed at several positions throughout the plate to monitor such variables as position effect, variability among wells, and timing difference between the addition of samples. Calculations for control charts should be done using absorbance values normalized by subtracting the cutoff value from the absorbance of the control. The net positive value (NPV) can then be monitored by plotting the results on quality control charts as described in the next section.

Monitoring EIA Performance with Quality Control Charts

Statistical Quality Control

Every assay run must contain the following controls; an in-house positive control, an in-house negative control, and the controls supplied by the manufacturer with each kit. It is important to understand the intended use of these different control materials. The manufacturer's controls are supplied to ensure that the kit is performing as described in the kit brochure. Values obtained for the positive and the negative control sera are used to calculate the positive/negative cutoff values and to evaluate the sensitivity (positive control) and specificity (negative control) of each assay run. The in-house positive and negative controls are used to ensure that the assay performs at the same level of sensitivity and specificitiy run to run, lot to lot, and year to year. The latter is accomplished by preparing large quantities of control materials and standardizing new lots by overlapping runs before the previous lot is exhausted.

The best way to use quality control charts is still being debated. Some authors favor a statistical approach similar to that used for clinical

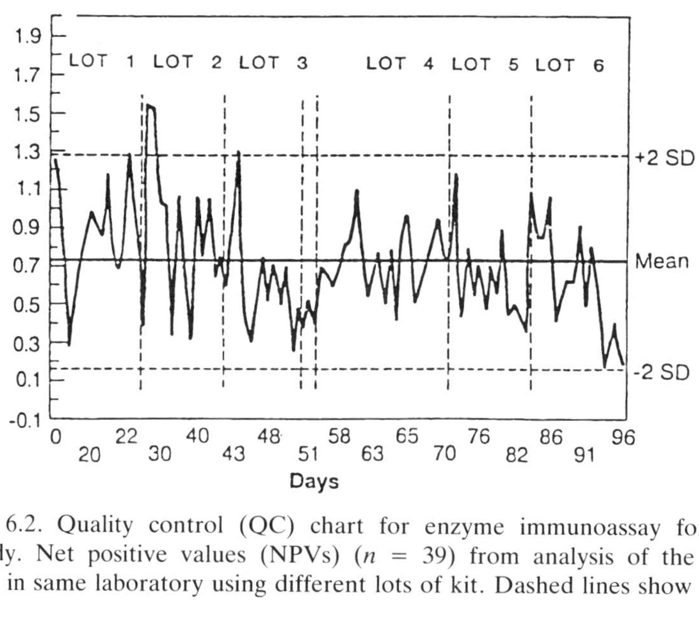

FIGURE 6.2. Quality control (QC) chart for enzyme immunoassay for HIV-1 antibody. Net positive values (NPVs) (n = 39) from analysis of the positive control in same laboratory using different lots of kit. Dashed lines show ±2 SD.

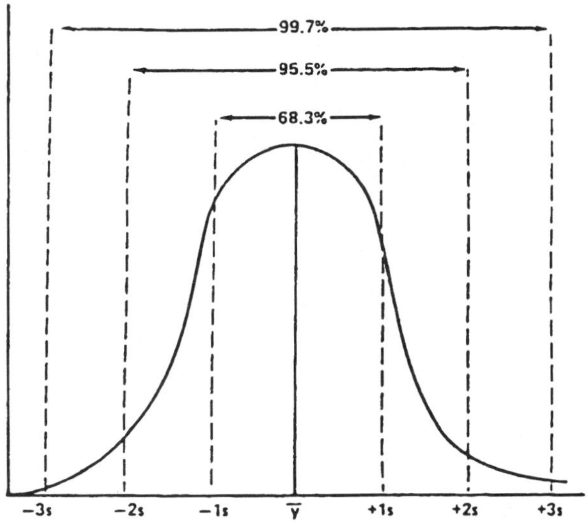

FIGURE 6.3. Fractional area under curve of normal (Gaussian) sample distribution.

chemistry analytes such as digoxin, thyroxine, or other hormones. These charts, called Shewhart or Levy–Jennings charts,[1,3] are prepared by analyzing duplicate samples of a control pool in at least 20 independent runs of the assay. Once this number is reached, the mean and standard deviation of the mean values are calculated. These values are used to produce a chart such as presented in Figure 6.2. This chart was drawn using the mean values of duplicate measurements of a HIV-1 antibody-positive control obtained from successive run with the FDA-licensed EIA.

Quality control charts prepared in this way are based on the assumption that data is normally distributed; this may not be the case. In a Gaussian or normal distribution, a fixed portion of the data falls within the interval given by the mean plus or minus (±) any multiple of the standard deviation, termed s. Figure 6.3 shows a Gaussian curve and the percentage of observations found within certain distances from the mean. For example, 68.3% of the observations will be within ±1.00 s of the mean; 95.5%, within ±2.00 s of the mean; and 99.7%, within ±3.00 s of the mean. It is common to talk about a 95% control and to estimate this by the mean ± 2.00 s, even though the correct multiplier would be 1.96 for a 95% limit. The same is true of the 99% control limit where ±3.00 s is often used when ±2.58 s is the correct value. Charts prepared as described offer visual evidence whether new measurements made on standard materials are from the distribution that we have observed previously in the laboratory over many runs. Variability in assay values is expected and inevitable. The analyst uses quality control charts to monitor and record the variability in the analytical process. Quality control charts present a history of the process in a diagrammatic form that is easy to follow.

Interpretation of Control Charts

The common statistical theory is that if a stable pattern continues to exist, in the long run approximately 99 of 100 future-run means will be between the upper and lower 99% control limits (mean ± 2.58 standard deviations, SD) and 19 of 20 will be between the upper and lower 95% control limit (mean ± 1.96 SD). This frequency (long run) is of interest, but you will be faced with deciding after each run whether your determinations are consistent with a stable pattern. If the mean should fall outside the 99% control level, what course of action should be taken? You are faced with two alternatives: (1) a stable pattern exists and you have just observed a rare event (it would occur 1 of 100 times in the long run), or (2) an unstable patteren has developed and the occurence is not just a rare event. Because the odds are against the rare event it would be sensible to check for condition 2. Suppose that a value fell outside the 95% control limits. Probability would say that this would occur 1 of 20 times when the system is stable. Two successive values, both above or below the 95% control limit, would indicate that the system is out of control, statistically speaking. On observing these signals all samples from these runs should be repeated.

While the statistical approach seems to satisfy our urge to be quantitative, it can be misleading and difficult to apply to the task of HIV antibody testing. If confidence intervals were calculated for the linear portion of Figure 6.1, it would be obvious that the relationship between antibody titer and absorbance is not linear and that the variability of the assay measured at various points along this curve is different. The variability at the high absorbance value is much greater than that observed at values close to the cutoff. Therefore, control materials giving high absorbance values may not reflect the stability of the assay at the cutoff. Further, EIA tests for HIV antibody are not intended to be quantitative. In fact, they are designed to tell you whether a sample is positive or negative for HIV antibody. Therefore, the only value that must be carefully controlled and stable is the cutoff absorbance. The application of a rigid statistical QC scheme might result in many false signals that a run is out of control when it is in fact functioning normally. Such runs would be repeated, resulting in extra work and expense.

Quality control charts can be used in a less rigid manner, without the use of control limits, to monitor the performance of HIV antibody EIAs. QC charts that plot the assay values of several controls on the same chart are very informative. In Figure 6.4, the NPV for the in-house low positive control and negative control is plotted simultaneously with the cutoff value of the assay. On the right edge of the chart, overlapping runs of

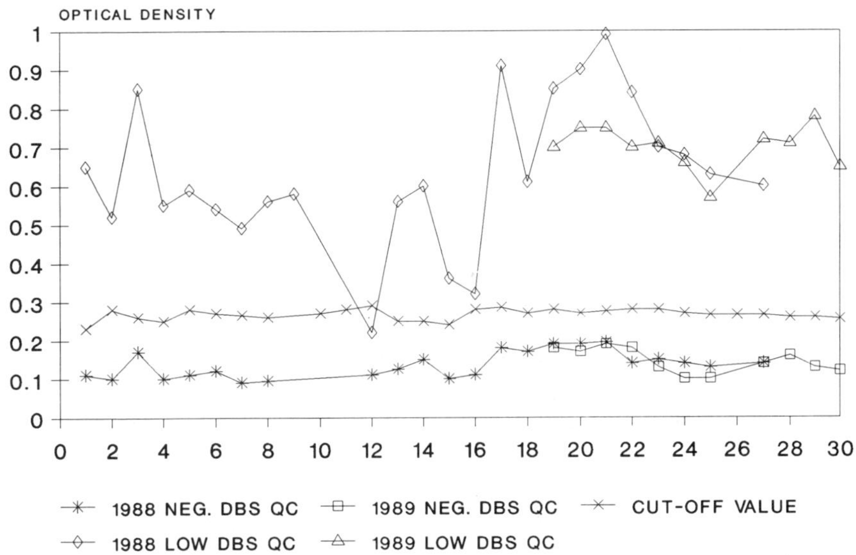

FIGURE 6.4. Net positive value (NPV) of in-house low positive control and negative are plotted with positive/negative cutoff value. Overlapping lines show how new lots are calibrated by overlapping runs using old and new lots of control sera.

new control pools are run with the current controls, indicating that new control materials are being introduced. This chart allows a visual presentation that permits trends in data to be detected early. Some of the sources of systematic error that can be detected are as follows:

1. Tendencies for all lines to move toward lower values could indicate deterioration of some assay component such as the conjugate or antigen-coated microplate.
2. Upward trends could indicate an unstable chromagen or instrument; for example, a plate reader or incubator.

Even though EIAs exhibit considerable variability, 15% to 20% among runs, within a given assay all absorbance values should vary in the same direction. If absorbances are lower than normal, all control values, including the cutoff, should be proportionally low to maintain the sensitivity of the assay. High background for negative samples should correspond to higher absorbances for the negative kit control. When control values vary independently, a random source of error should be suspected, such as pipetting, improper mixing of reagents, or improper plate washing. Such random errors usually can be eliminated by examining one's technique. Careful pipetting of samples and assay components can dramatically improve the reproducibility of the assay values and tighten the scatter of control points.

Charts that monitor the variability of the kit controls as well as the in-house controls permit changes in the assay introduced by the manufacturer to be identified. For example, if only kit controls are run and monitored, a shift downward in kit sensitivity could be masked by increasing the potency of kit controls. This would be immediately detected by a chart that monitors the in-house and kit positive control (Figure 6.5). Such a situation would produce a downward shift in values for the in-house control while the kit control values remain at their usual levels.

H. G. Wells, in his essay "Mind at the End of Its Tether," said, "We live in reference to past events." It is unlikely that Wells was thinking of quality control when he wrote these words but he does describe the principle of QC charts. These charts allow us to monitor the performance of an assay over time using the same pool of control materials. When the values produced by as assay deviates from the norm established by our past experience, we should look for the source of the variability. Furthermore, within a given population one would soon learn how many positives to expect in a given run, or how many low positives that do not repeat normally occurs within a given plate. Sudden or even gradual shifts in the expected can reflect changes in the population or more usually changes in the test system.

Quality Control of Western Blot

Quality control of the western blot test for HIV antibody is more difficult than that for EIA, primarily because the QC recommendations must be a compromise between what is scientifically satisfying and what is economically feasible. Commercial western blots cost between $18 and $45 per test for the FDA-licensed reagents. In each assay run, it is necessary to run strongly positive, weakly positive, and negative controls supplied by the manufacturer. In a run of 27 strips, the number of strips in the Biotech/Du Pont/Ortho kit, approximately 10% of the reagents are used for quality control. It is difficult to recommend that additional QC samples be run because it is doubtful that they would significantly improve the quality of the test results. Occasional use of in-house positive controls may be helpful to demonstrate that the reactivity against various proteins is consistent in intensity and position among various lots of reagents.

It is important, however, that the QC samples from the manufacturer be carefully examined and the results appropriately analyzed. The strongly positive control is used primarily to demonstrate that the antigen strips contain all the proteins required to test for HIV infection. It also provides a reference for the position of these bands on the strips. Runs in which critical bands are missing must be rejected. The weakly reactive control is a reference for the intensity. In both licensed kits, Ortho and

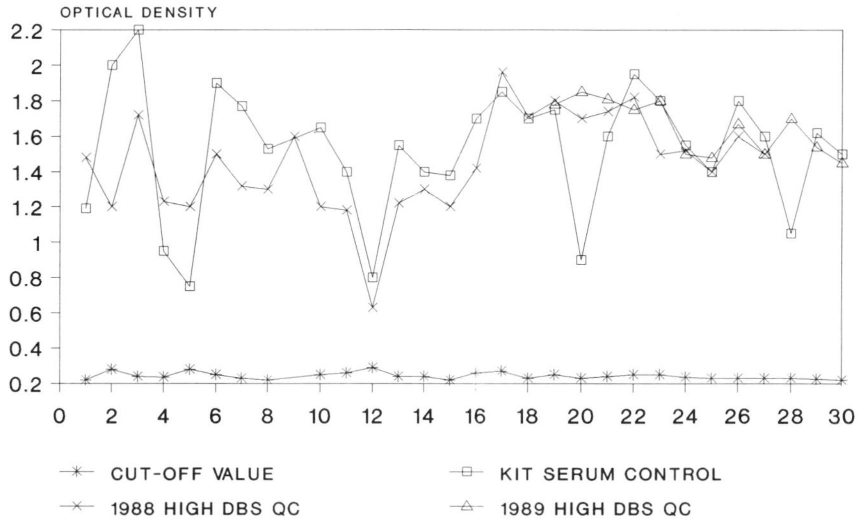

FIGURE 6.5. Net positive value (NPV) of kit positive control sera is plotted with positive control.

Bio-Rad, the bands of test samples are assigned a reactivity score based on a comparison with a band on the weakly reactive control. These reference bands should be carefully examined to ensure that their intensity has not significantly increased or decreased for a particular run. Reference bands that are weaker than normal increase the sensitivity of the tests and could cause bands to be scored as reactive (+) that normally would be $\pm$. This could increase the number of indeterminate results. Reference bands that are stronger than normal decreases the sensitivity of a test. Sera that normally would be positive may become indeterminate. Negative control strips should show *no* bands. Presence of bands on the negative control strip could result from splashover from adjacent wells or, more seriously, indicate deterioration of the kit.

Proficiency Testing

Every laboratory performing HIV testing should be enrolled in one or more proficiency testing program. Such programs are available from the College of American Pathologists, the American Association of Bioanalysts, and the Centers for Disease Control. These programs permit laboratories to be tested to see how well they are performing in relation to other laboratories that use the same and different tests. Unfortunately, proficiency testing panels are not very challenging and usually detect only gross deficiencies in laboratory performance. Certainly such programs are no substitute for rigorous QC programs within each laboratory.

Other Quality Control Requirements

Specimen Collection

All assays require that the proper specimen be collected and handled in the prescribed manner. The manufacturers' instructions as contained in the kit brochure should be carefully studied and all recommendations followed. Some important points in specimen collection follow:

1. Should plasma or serum be collected? If plasma is to be tested, the anticoagulant could be important for some tests.
2. Does hemolyzed, lipemic, or icteric samples interfere with the tests to be performed?
3. Does the test require fresh samples? Certain assays (Recombigen Latex Agglutination) require samples that have never been frozen. Other tests work perfectly well with frozen samples.

Equipment

Equipment should be subjected to daily monitoring and routine maintenance.

1. Temperature of refrigerators, freezers, waterbaths, and incubators must be checked daily.
2. Microplate readers (spectrophotomers) should be periodically cleaned and calibrated. Linearity of microplate readers should be checked. Microplate readers are probably the most neglected instruments in the laboratory, mainly because the manufacturers do not emphasize the necessity of preventive maintenance and calibration to their customers. However, when asked, most manufacturers can provide protocols and standards for these calibrations.
3. Microplate washers must be subjected to a rigorous daily regimen of cleaning and when necessary, adjustment. Washers must be flushed and disinfected, and waste materials carefully disinfected and discarded. Washers are especially subject to corrosion because of the high salt content of the buffers that they dispense. This is further aggravated by poor design, which allows spilled wash solution to reach the internal parts of the machine.
4. Finally, pipets should be periodically cleaned and calibrated. Even the most careful technologist will eventually draw liquid into the pipet. Certain companies will provide maintenance and calibration service at your laboratory for approximatly $30 per pipet. Each technologist should be carefully instructed in proper pipetting techniques and be required to demonstrate proficiency before allowed to begin actual testing.

Unreliable HIV antibody test results reported to the physician can be extremely detrimental to the physical and mental well-being of the patient. To recognize inaccurate assay results, therefore, a well-conceived and well-executed program of quality control is essential. In addition, the laboratorian must also understand the complex physical and immunological principles involved in the assay. Through this understanding, signals of inaccuracy generated by quality control will be recognized, the source of inaccuracy identified, and the appropriate corrective action taken.

References

1. Westgard JO, Barry PL. Cost-Effective Quality Control: Managing the Quality and Productivity of Analytical Processes. Washington, DC: American Association for Clinical Chemistry Press, 1986:17.
2. Kudlac J, Hanan S, McKee GL. Development of quality control procedures for the human immunodeficiency virus type 1 antibody enzyme-linked immunosorbent assay. J Clin Microbiol 1989;27:1303–1306.
3. George JR, Palmer DF, Cavallaro JJ, Wagner WM. Principles of Radioimmunoassay: Immunology Series No. 12. Public Health Service, U.S. Department of Health and Human Services, 1984.

7
Direct Detection of Human Immunodeficiency Virus Infection Using the Polymerase Chain Reaction

GERALD SCHOCHETMAN and JOHN J. SNINSKY

Although infectious viral particles of human immunodeficiency virus (HIV) encapsidate single-stranded RNA (ssRNA) as the genetic information, the viral life cycle includes a compulsory conversion to double-stranded DNA (dsDNA), termed the provirus, which becomes integrated into the host cell's chromosomes. The integrated provirus remains associated with the cellular chromosomal DNA for the life of the infected cell. Further, the integrated provirus can either actively transcribe the genes for the structural proteins of the virus, which results in the assembly and release of infectious virions, or, by selective transcription of only the complex array of viral regulatory genes, remain transcriptionally constrained and thereby not release viral particles. The latter condition is frequently referred to as the "latent state." Because proviral DNA is present regardless of the transcriptional state of the cell, early efforts targeted to direct detection of the virus used proviral DNA as a template.

Because of the low frequency of HIV-1-infected peripheral blood mononuclear cells (PBMCs) in a seropositive person,[1] conventional molecular biology techniques[2] were not sensitive enough to routinely detect and characterize HIV proviral DNA directly from a patient's lymphocytes. Therefore, HIV proviral DNA must first be amplified to detectable levels using the polymerase chain reaction (PCR). Before PCR, successful direct detection of HIV-1 required culturing the virus. However, the ability of PCR to amplify HIV sequences orders of magnitude in vitro obviated the need to propagate the virus for direct detection.

In the study of HIV infection and AIDS, PCR has demonstrated both clinical and research utility for (i) the direct detection and quantitation of HIV DNA and RNA from cells of infected persons; (ii) detecting infected persons during the window period (i.e., before the generation of HIV-specific antibodies); (iii) resolving the infection status of individuals with an indeterminate western blot; (iv) screening of neonates for HIV infection; (v) distinguishing HIV-1 from HIV-2 infections; and (vi) defining the patterns of transmission and evolution of the virus throughout the population.

PCR Methodology

The PCR process was originally developed as a technique for the in vitro amplification of targeted DNA sequences.[3–6] For PCR, sample preparation has employed the separation of the mononuclear from the polymorphonuclear cells of the blood using a Ficoll-hypaque gradient. Following preparation of the peripheral blood mononuclear cells (PBMCs), the cells are incubated with nonionic detergents and finally treated with proteinase K. Heat treatment at 95°C for 15 minutes is used to inactivate the proteinase K; the resulting DNA preparation is ready for PCR. Usually 1 μg of DNA (equivalent to about 150,000 mononuclear cells; Table 7.1) is used per PCR reaction. PCR is a repetitive process consisting of three distinct steps (Figure 7.1): (i) denaturation of dsDNA, (ii) annealing of specific primers, and (iii) extension of annealed primers. Because DNA is complementary and antiparallel, ssDNA can also serve as a templete for amplification. When amplification of a specific RNA sequence is required, a DNA copy of the RNA sequence is produced using the enzyme reverse transcriptase before PCR amplification of the resulting DNA.[7,8] Following the PCR process, a variety of techniques can be used to detect

TABLE 7.1. Numbers to consider for HIV infection.

5.6 liters of blood in 70-kg person
500,000 white blood cells/65 μl whole blood
White Blood Cells
350,000 polymorphonuclear cells (70%)
150,000 mononuclear cells (30%)
Mononuclear Cells
15,000 monocytes (10%)
15,000 large granular lymphocytes (LGL) (10%)
15,000 B cells (10%)
105,000 T cells (70%)
T Cells
37,000 T8 (suppressor) cells (35%)
68,000 T4 (helper) cells (65%)

TABLE 7.2. Reaction parameters to be evaluated for efficient PCR.

Annealing temperature and time
Denaturation temperature and time
Taq DNA polymerase addition at elevated temperature
Enzyme concentration
$MgCl_2$ concentration
Primer concentration
Cosolvents

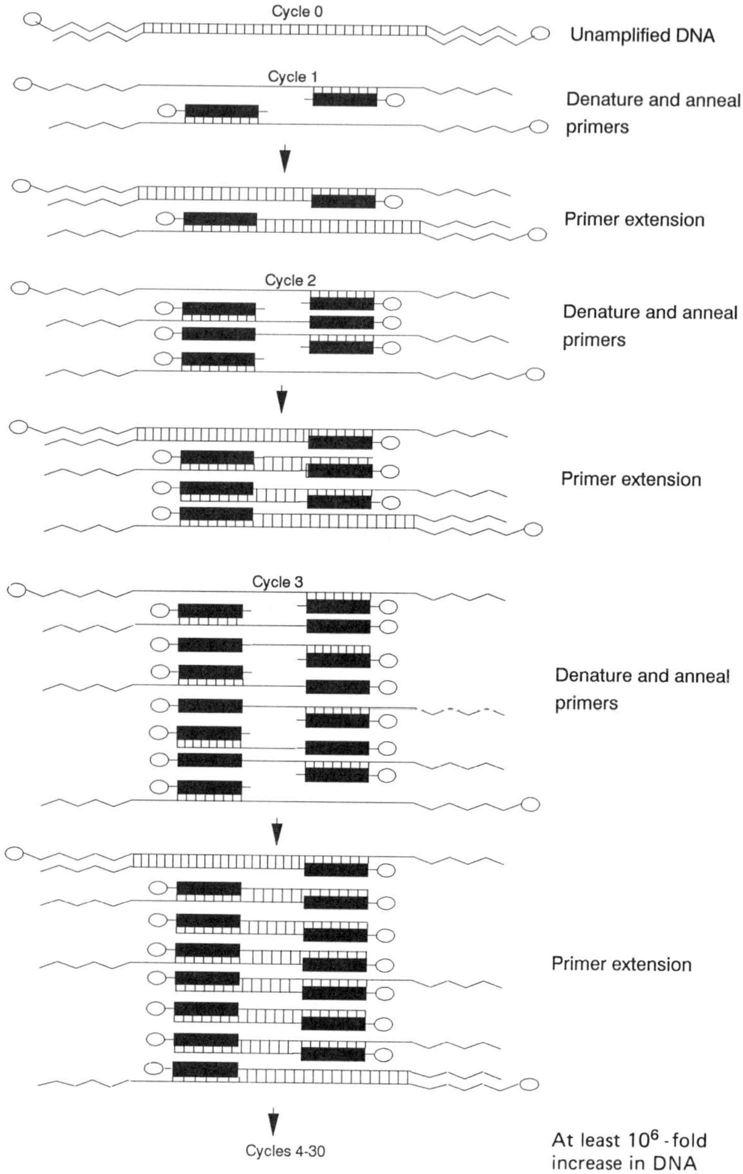

FIGURE 7.1. Polymerase chain reaction (PCR) is a repetitive process including denaturation of double-stranded DNA (dsDNA), annealing of primers, and extension of bound primers. One PCR cycle requires about 3 minutes; cycle is repeated, usually 25–35 times. dsDNA is first heated to 95–100°C to separate strands of duplex. During subsequent annealing phase, oligonucleotide primers hybridize to dissociated HIV DNA. Each primer is complementary to one original DNA strand, either the 5′ or 3′ side of sequence of interest. Following annealing, a thermostable DNA polymerase from *Thermus aquaticus* (*Taq*) is used to catalyze the synthesis of new strands of DNA that are complementary to intervening sequences primed by opposing oligonucleotide primers.

the amplified DNA sequences. Although the amplified DNA is of a defined size and can sometimes be visualized after gel electrophoresis, this method cannot provide definitive identification of the product. The confirmation of amplification of HIV DNA includes hybridization of a portion of the amplified DNA to a synthetic DNA probe that is complementary to a portion of the amplified DNA sequence. The probe can be labeled by a variety of means, isotopic (radioactive) or nonisotopic (colorimetric or chemiluminescent) (Figures 7.2–7.4).

Direct Detection of HIV Proviral Sequences

PCR has proven to be a powerful technique for diagnosing HIV infections. It has been successfully used for direct detection of HIV-1 proviral DNA sequences in PBMCs of seropositive persons[9–12] and to detect HIV-1 DNA in cells from seropositive subjects who were negative by virus coculture.[9] Studies have also demonstrated that PCR has simplified the ability of researchers to directly clone and sequence HIV-1 DNA[13–15] and HIV-1 cellular RNA.[7] HIV sequences obtained by this method more accurately reflect the repertoire of viral sequences actually present in a patient.[14] This is possible because PCR does not require virus isolation, which leads to the selection of only a subset of the HIV strains that are present in any particular patient.[14,15]

PCR has been used to establish that virtually all antibody-positive persons are infected with HIV, lending further proof that HIV is the

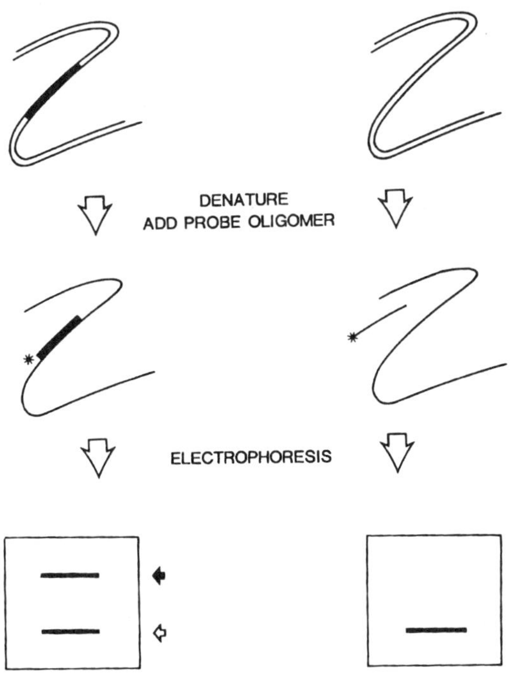

FIGURE 7.2. Detection of amplified DNA: hybridization of portion of amplified DNA product to radioactive ^{32}P-labeled synthetic probe complementary to portion of amplified sequences, followed by gel analysis and autoradiography.

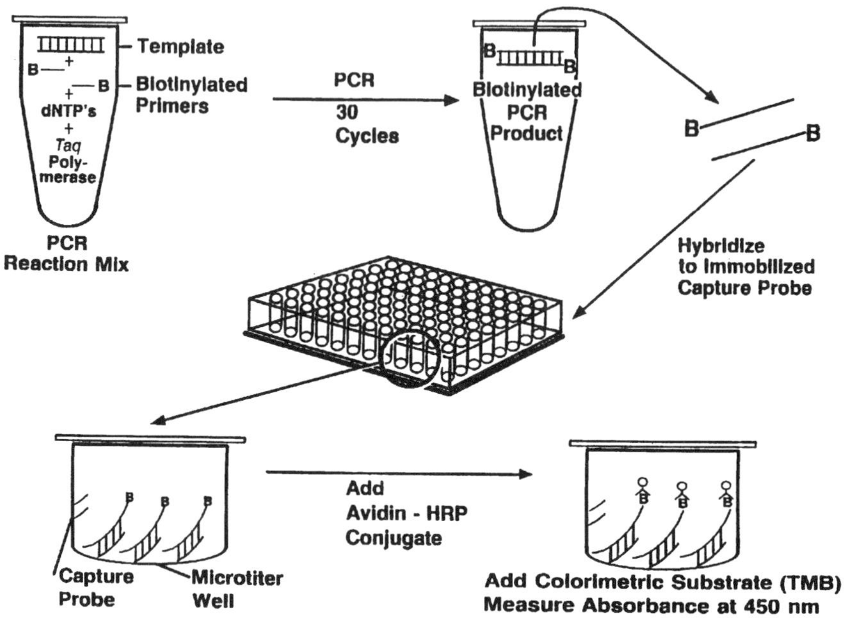

FIGURE 7.3. Detection of amplified DNA: biotinylated primers generate tagged amplified DNA product that is then hybridized to immobilized probe complementary to portion of amplified sequences, followed by incubation with avidin conjugated to horseradish peroxidase. This standard EIA format in a microplate yields a colorimetric readout for positive samples (C. Silver, M. Sulzinski, E. Dragon, and M. Longiaru, personal communication).

causative agent of AIDS.[16] This large-scale study involved testing of peripheral blood mononuclear cells obtained from 409 individuals who were HIV antibody positive. The group consisted of 56 who had AIDS, 88 who had AIDS-related complex (ARC), and 265 who were asymptomatic. In addition, blood samples from 131 persons who were HIV antibody negative were also examined. All samples from the 56 AIDS patients, 87 of the 88 ARC patients (99%), and 259 of the 265 asymptomatic but HIV antibody-positive persons (98%) tested positive for virus by culture, by PCR, or by both analyses; in contrast, none of the 131 HIV-1 antibody-negative persons was positive for virus by culture or by PCR.

Quantitation of HIV Proviral Sequences

Because the amount of the original target DNA can be quantitated by PCR, the technique can be used to measure the number of infected cells[17–19] or to quantitate the amount of cell-free virus in the plasma

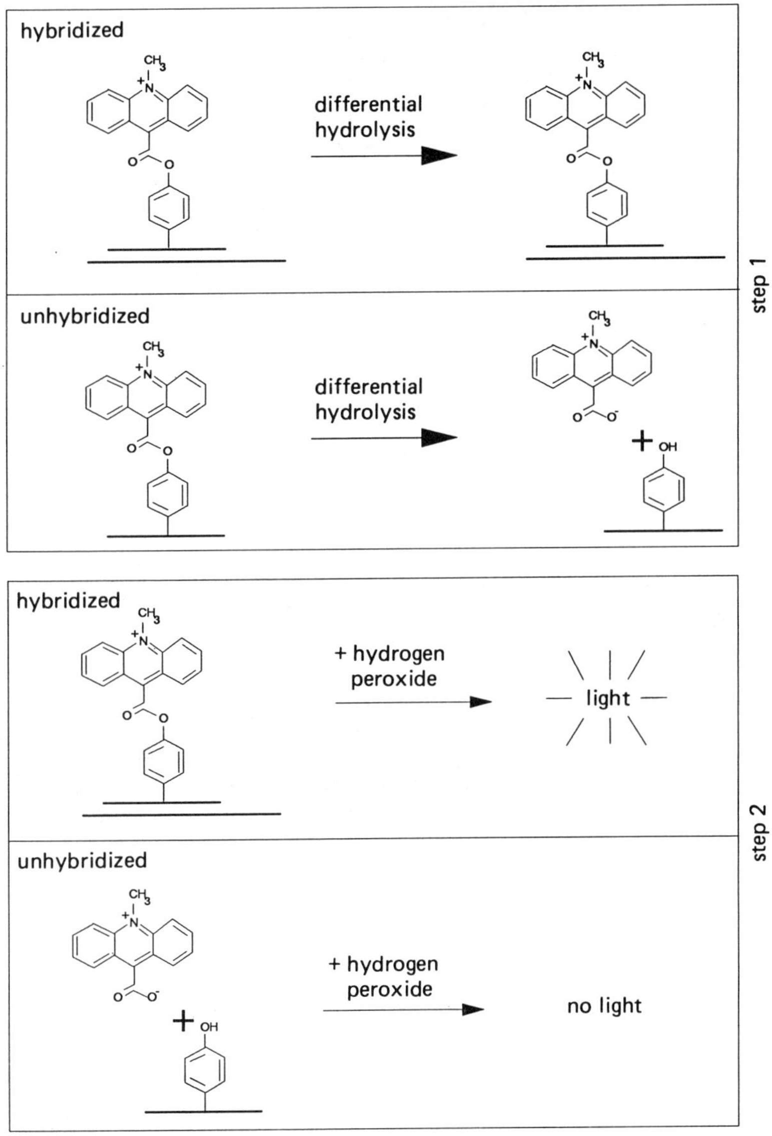

FIGURE 7.4. Detection of amplified DNA: hybridization of portion of amplified DNA product to acridinium-labeled synthetic probe complementary to portion of amplified sequences is followed by differential alkaline hydrolysis (Step 1). Acridinium attached to hybridized probe is relatively resistant to alkaline hydrolysis and can chemiluminesce after oxidation by addition of hydrogen peroxide (Step 2). In contrast, acridinium attached to unhybridized probe is highly sensitive to alkaline degradation and loses ability to chemiluminescence almost immediately.

(viremia) in a patient. A quantitative assay for proviral HIV-1 would be important for the evaluation of new drugs and vaccines or for monitoring disease progression. Quantitation of viral load in infected persons has been performed with varying success, by limiting dilution culture methods in which culture supernatants were tested for the presence of HIV-1 *gag* protein (p24) or the presence of viral reverse transcriptase activity.[20,21] Virus culture is expensive and time consuming, requires handling of large volumes of infectious material, and has not always been reliable. By amplifying a dilution series of known amounts of HIV DNA (e.g., a plasmid containing a full-length copy of HIV-1 DNA, or DNA from a cell line containing one integrated copy of HIV-1 per cell), it is possible to quantify the virus burden in a person by determining the number of HIV proviral copies per given number of cells in a patient.[17–19,22–26] To ensure the biosafe use of a full-length proviral DNA standard, a replication-deficient HIV-1 proviral DNA has been developed.[27] A cell line, ACH2, which contains one integrated copy of HIV-1 and produces a noninfectious HIV has also been developed.[28] Methods have also been developed for the quantitation of specific RNAs by the PCR technique.[29–31] Recently, a rapid and quantitative detection procedure was developed using a non-isotopic chemiluminescent DNA probe.[18] The total time for PCR amplification and DNA probing, using this new technique, was about 4 hours. Thus, detection and quantitation of HIV DNA could be achieved in 1 to 1.5 days from the time of receipt of the blood sample.

PCR has been used by a number of investigators to determine the relation between infected cell burden and immunologic status in persons with asymptomatic and symptomatic HIV infection.[19,24–26] In those studies, lysates of patient PBMCs were serially diluted, amplified, and detected with a radiolabeled probe. The signal intensity from each amplification was compared with PCR performed on serial dilutions of the plasmid containing the HIV-1 genome or the ACH2 cell line that contains one integrated copy of HIV-1 per cell. The results of those studies demonstrated that there was a significant increase in viral burden per constant $CD4^+$ cells in patients as they progressed to clinical disease. There was also a concomitant quantitative depletion of $CD4^+$ cells, in contrast with the stable viral burden and the maintenance of a relatively constant level of $CD4^+$ cells in patients who were clinically stable.[24] The number of HIV-infected cells can be calculated from the number of proviral copies because it has been estimated that there is approximately one proviral copy per cell.[25] These results can be compared to the number of cells producing virus in asymptomatic versus symptomatic persons as determined by limiting dilution cultures.[20,21]

From this type of analysis it can be estimated that approximately 10% of the infected cells in asymptomatic persons are actively expressing virus, compared to about 100% of the infected cells in symptomatic persons. These results indicate that not only do the number of infected cells increase substantially, but that the proportion of infected cells actively expressing HIV increases substantially as patients move from an asymptomatic to a symptomatic state. These results are consistent with a direct and probable causal relation between increase in viral burden, and immunosuppression and disease, presumably because of the increase in HIV expression leading to cell destruction.

Latent HIV-1 infection can be differentiated from active viral transcription[7,8,32] because HIV-specific RNA sequences can be detected in cells of infected persons by amplifying cDNA copies of reverse-transcribed cellular RNA. This assay was capable of detecting HIV RNA in 1 infected cell among 10^6 uninfected cells.[7] Direct comparison of the presence of detectable HIV serum antigen, with HIV RNA expression in the same patients,[7] demonstrated that RNA PCR was more sensitive than serum antigen detection (i.e., all patients that were antigen positive were HIV RNA positive, but all patients that were HIV RNA positive were not antigen positive).

Viral Infection and Seroconversion

Various reports have indicated that in some persons HIV can be detected by virus isolation or by antigen detection before seroconversion.[33–37] Other studies have reported that HIV-1 proviral DNA can be detected in PBMCs before seroconversion.[38–41] Preliminary replication of one of these studies[41] has not confirmed the original results (unpublished data) and merits additional investigation. Persons who have been followed prospectively after exposure to HIV-1 have generally seroconverted within 6 months.[42] However, cases of positive antigen reactions for as long as 14 months without detectable antibody have also been reported.[35,39] To define the length of time from infection to development of detectable levels of HIV antibodies, a study was undertaken of 26 homosexual men and 11 men with hemophilia pre- and post seroconversion.[42] PBMCs from these men were analyzed for HIV-1 DNA by PCR using primers from two distinct regions of the viral genome. Using a Markov statistical model, the median time from infection with HIV-1 to seroconversion was estimated to be within 3 months and that 95% of all persons who become infected would seroconvert within 6 months. These results indicated that prolonged periods of latent infection without detectable antibody probably are rare.

Resolving Persons with Indeterminate Western Blots

PCR has been used to determine whether apparently healthy persons who have had repeatedly reactive EIAs and an indeterminate western blot for HIV antibody are infected with HIV-1.[43] A total of 99 volunteer blood donors in a low-risk area of the United States with such a serologic outcome were coded and tested for the presence of HIV by culture and by PCR. Of the 99 blood donors, 98 had no reported risk factors for HIV-1 infection; 1 donor had used intravenous drugs. After a median of 14 months from the time of the initial serologic tests, 65 donors (66%) were still repeatedly reactive for HIV-1 on at least one immunoassay. In 91 donors (92%), the western blot results were still indeterminate. None of the 99 donors had evidence of either HIV infection as determined by both culture or by PCR. These results demonstrate that persons at low risk (e.g., volunteer blood donors) for HIV infection and who have persistent indeterminate HIV-1 western blots are rarely infected with HIV-1.

HIV Typing

HIV-1 and HIV-2 share partial but significant serologic cross-reactivity between their *gag* (core) proteins whereas cross-reactive antibodies to the *env* (envelope) proteins are thought to be considerably less common.[44] Recently, there have been reports of persons who possess antibodies reactive against the *gag*, *pol*, and *env* proteins of both HIV-1 and HIV-2.[44–48] Serologically, it has been difficult to determine whether this dual reactivity resulted from a single HIV infection generating a broad immune response to determinants common to both viruses, an infection with a recombinant or third virus containing determinants of both HIV-1 and HIV-2, or a true mixed infection with both viruses in the same person. In regions where HIV-1 but not HIV-2 is highly endemic (e.g., the United States), it would be unlikely to find a person infected with both viruses. However, in certain areas of West Africa where HIV-1 and HIV-2 are both prevalent, the probability of finding a person infected with both viruses would be much higher.

PCR has been successfully used as an adjunct to serologic testing to determine if a patient is infected with HIV-1 or HIV-2.[48] PCR has been used to confirm the first case of HIV-2 infection in a person living in the United States[49] and has been also used to confirm the first case of a mixed HIV-1 and HIV-2 infection in the same person.[48] This latter person was seroreactive by whole-virus EIAs, type-specific peptide EIAs, and western blots for both viruses, and contained proviral sequences of both HIV-1 and HIV-2 as determined by PCR.

HIV Infection in Newborns

The fact that no more than one-third of infants born to HIV-1-seropositive mothers become infected and the presence of maternal antibodies to HIV-1 in the newborn makes diagnosis of HIV-1 infection difficult. PCR has been used successfully to diagnosis HIV-1 infection by detecting HIV-1 DNA during the neonatal period (first 28 days of life) in those infants born to HIV-seropositive mothers who develop a severe and rapid course of disease.[50,51] The PCR has also detected virtually all HIV-infected children who are in the postneonatal period, usually a few months old.[50–52] Those HIV-infected infants born to seropositive mothers who develop a less severe and slow course of disease become HIV PCR positive by 4–6 months. However, diagnosis of HIV-1 infection during the neonatal period and assessment of disease outcome in seropositive infants[50,51] is essential for identifying infants that might benefit from early therapeutic intervention[51,53] (see also Chapter 11 for a more complete description).

Use of PCR to Monitor for Drug-Resistant HIV

The reverse transcriptase inhibitor 3′-azido-3′-deoxythymidine (AZT or zidovudine), has demonstrated clinical utility for the treatment of AIDS and ARC. Specifically, this therapeutic strategy has been shown to extend life expectancy and to lower the frequency and severity of opportunistic infections. The initially reported isolates with reduced sensitivity in vitro to this nucleoside analogue,[54] cultured from patients receiving zidovudine, were subsequently found to harbor specific mutations within the coding sequence for the HIV reverse transcriptase.[55] Although the most resistant isolates have four amino acid substitutions (e.g., positions 67, 70, 215, and 219), isolates that have a subset of these four mutations are less resistant to the drug. Recently, a "nested" or "double" PCR procedure was developed[56] to detect the common mutations found in residue 215 (e.g., conversion of the threonine codon to one for either tyrosine or phenylalanine requires a two-base change). Under modified conditions,[57] PCR can also be used to selectively amplify sequences varying in a single nucleotide; therefore, the other codon changes should be amenable to similar analysis. The role these mutations play in the declining efficacy of zidovudine after protracted periods of treatment remains unclear, but rapid diagnostic procedures for their detection will assist in resolving their contribution.

Analytical Sensitivity and Specificity

The PCR has the greatest analytical sensitivity of any procedure that has been used in the diagnostic arena. Single molecule detection has been reported by numerous laboratories. This exquisite analytical sensitivity does not necessarily translate into diagnostic sensitivity with the ultimate clinical utility. The procedure does not have an intrinsic analytic or diagnostic sensitivity and specificity. The diagnostic sensitivity and specificity is inextricably linked to the laboratories performing the procedure. As a result, the confidence in the reported results is directly proportional to the experience and critical interpretive criteria used by the laboratories performing the assay. Multiple parameters have been shown to dramatically affect the overall analytical sensitivity and correspondingly its diagnostic sensitivity.

Factors that have been demonstrated to affect overall amplification efficiency beyond the obvious contribution of the selected primers and probes for amplification and detection, respectively, include the concentration of the various reagents and the thermocycling profiles used for amplification (see Table 7.2). Thus, as with other diagnostic assays, the use of well-characterized controls to monitor inter- and intra-assay variability is essential. The introduction of the use of PCR for the detection of HIV has resulted in several controversial reports that run counter to the experience of others in the diagnostic community carrying out this procedure. PCR data in the absence of patient follow-up and supporting results from more established procedures, such as the FDA-approved EIAs or viral culture by an experienced laboratory, should be viewed with caution.

Similar to other diagnostic assays, the application of PCR to the detection of HIV proviral DNA has resulted in false-positives and false-negatives. False-positives have been demonstrated to result from (i) cross-contamination of a negative sample from a positive sample, (ii) contamination of clinical samples or the reagents for amplification with recombinant plasmids or phage harboring the entire or portions of the HIV proviral genome, and (iii) "carryover" of PCR products from previous positive reactions. The latter is usually the reason for false-positives because of the number of copies generated by the PCR (e.g., 10^6–10^{12}). Higuchi and Kwok[58] have recommended specific precautions to follow to minimize this type of contamination (see *Carryover*, following). In addition, two laboratories[59,60] have described the use of deoxyuridine triphosphate (dUTP) instead of deoxythymidine triphosphate (dTTP) and the other three conventional deoxynucleoside triphosphates in PCR and pretreatment of all reactions with uracil DNA glycosylase (UNG) to eliminate or "sterilize" errant PCR products as templates for the amplification (Figure 7.5). Just as PCR harnesses the replication capacity of cells, this procedure exploits the restriction/modification and excision/repair systems of cells. Because PCR products containing deoxyuridine hybridize as efficiently as deoxythymidine-containing PCR products, and can be cloned and sequenced, this procedural modification promises to increase the reliability of positive results from a large number of laboratories.

False-negatives have been attributed to compromised analytic sensitivity because of insufficient specificity as the result of either less than optimal amplification conditions or the selection of primers and probes that do not readily recognize different sequence variants.[57]

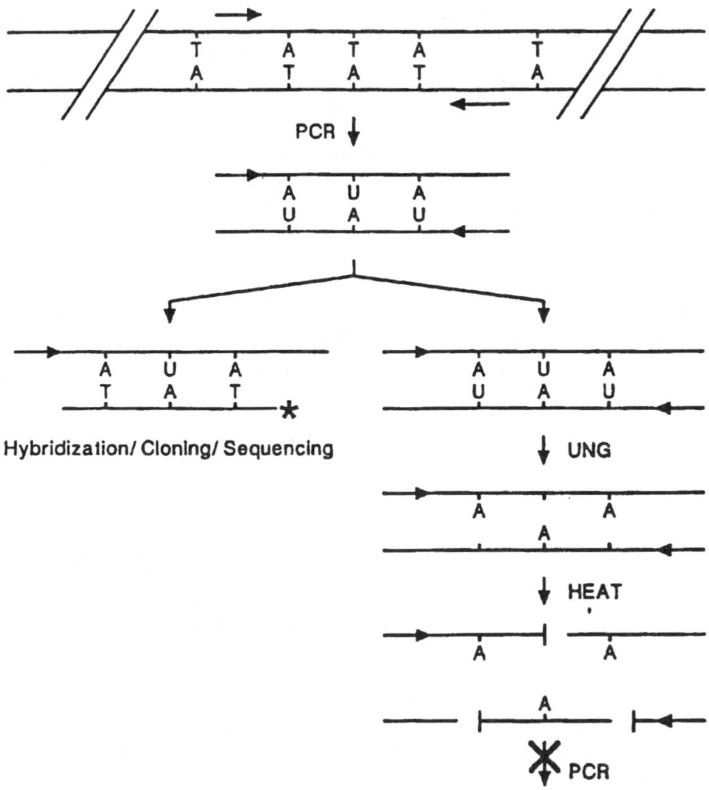

FIGURE 7.5. Use of deoxyuridine triphosphate (dUTP) and uracil DNA glycosylase (UNG) to eliminate errant PCR products as templates for subsequent amplifications leading to false-positives.

As with all diagnostic assays, replication is an important element, so that one may be confident that the results are reproducible. Samples that have disparate results in duplicate, not unlike the discordant EIA assays, can be caused by signals at the cutoff for positivity or by sample mixup. Stochastically, a sample must contain five copies of HIV template to have a 99% likelihood of being reproducibly positive. If there are fewer than an average of five copies in a sample, the reactions may appear irreproducible due to sampling bias.

Recently, a multicenter, blinded proficiency trial using 105 HIV-1 seronegative, culture-negative samples from low-risk blood donors and 99 HIV-1 seropositive and culture-positive samples was completed.[61] The five laboratories participating in the study had significant experience with PCR; however, the procedure and interpretive criteria varied somewhat and only one of the multiple primer pairs was used in common. The average sensitivity for the laboratories was 99.0%; the average specificity was 94.7%. One laboratory achieved 100% sensitivity and specificity. The overall false-positive, false-negative, and indeterminate rates were 1.8, 0.8, and 1.9%, respectively. This study demonstrated that PCR is a highly sensitive and specific assay for HIV-1 proviral DNA but that rigorous procedural and critical testing algorithms are required. Further, the two primer pair systems targeted to the *gag* gene showed 100% sensitivity and specificity. This observation suggests that the inability to detect all samples known to contain HIV-1 proviral DNA at the requisite level with different primer pairs may result from a laboratory's experimental performance rather than a viral sequence variant incapable of amplification.

The lack of concordance between duplicate samples may be caused by sample mixup. Resolution of sample mixup when using serologic assays is difficult. Often, the sample is either rerun or another sample is taken for analysis. However, PCR assays for HIV allow for simple resolution, particularly if amplification of the histocompatibility region is used as a control for the number of cells examined and amplification integrity of the sample. The pioneering PCR studies of Erlich and colleagues[62] on HLA genotyping were later exploited for HIV[63] to demonstrate that due to the polymorphic nature of the region between the HLA DQ alpha DNA primers used, samples from different individuals could be discerned because of the differential hybridization of HLA sequence-specific probes[64] (Figure 7.6).

Laboratories using PCR for HIV detection in PBMCs of infected individuals often use multiple primer pairs because of the sequence heterogeneity of viral variants. Thirteen of 18 published studies demonstrated concordance between the primer-pair-probe systems used on the same sample. Six of the 13 studies used the SK38–39 primer/SK19 probe system and the SK145–101 primer/SK102 probe system for examining more than 1,000 specimens. Of the seven remaining studies, four used the SK38–39 system compared to an additional primer pair-probe system.

The five additional published studies showed discordance between or among primer pairs with the same sample. Reasons for the disagreement between results from different primer pair systems on the same sample may be multifold and include: (i) sequence heterogeneity obviating amplification of one of the two systems, (ii) differential analytical sensitivity of the two systems, (iii) sample bias due to copy numbers below five, (iv) carryover of products from previous reactions, or (v) deletion of the entire or a portion of the region recognized by one of the primer pair systems. The use of long primers (25 or more bases), the presence of a T residue at the 3′ terminus, and lower annealing temperatures have been shown to decrease the likelihood that sequence heterogeneity among viral variants will lead to discordant results. When performing studies with multiple primer pairs, it is important to ensure that each system has equivalent analytical sensitivity. This can be accomplished by using a common control, such as a plasmid containing the HIV genome, to avoid

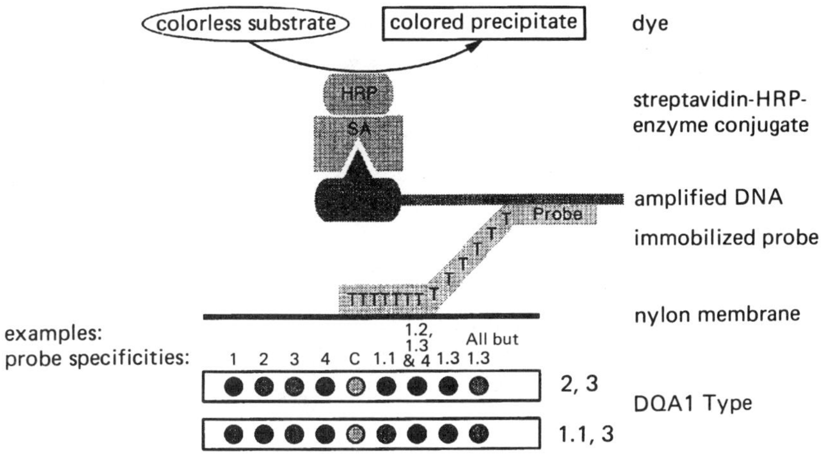

FIGURE 7.6. Reverse dot blot hybridization with sequence-specific probes to rapidly and precisely type HLA DQ alpha class II polymorphism shown in schematic diagram of immobilized oligonucleotide probe detection of amplified DNA. Sequence-specific probe is "tailed" with a dT (deoxythymidine) homopolymer and immobilized on a solid support. Amplified PCR product, which has incorporated biotinylated primer, hybridizes to probe. After washing away unbound DNA and primers, biotinylated, amplified DNA binds an avidin horseradish peroxidase conjugate. Enzyme then converts colorless dye into colored precipitate. Format shown is for detecting specific alleles in samples of amplified DQ alpha DNA from heterozygous individuals.

conflicting results. Careful examination of the studies reporting discordant results indicate that the two most likely reasons for the discordancy are the use of short primers (18–20 bases) and the use of conditions known not to be optimal for analytical sensitivity.

Carryover

As mentioned earlier, considerable care must be taken to avoid carryover of DNA from one tube to another to prevent false-positives.[58] Because amplified sequences are present in large numbers, carryover of minute quantities of amplified DNA can lead to significant false-positive problems. The following is a list of procedures that should minimize carryover.

Physical Separation of Pre-PCR and Post-PCR Reactions

To prevent carryover, a separate room or containment unit, such as a biosafety cabinet, should be used for setting up amplification reactions. A separate set of supplies and pipettes should be kept in this area and should be used only for setting up PCR reactions. Care must be taken to ensure that amplified DNA is not brought into this area. Reagents, devices, and supplies should never be taken and returned from an area where PCR analyses are being performed.

Aliquot Reagents

Reagents should be aliquoted to minimize the number of repeated samplings. All reagents used in the PCR process must be prepared, aliquoted, and stored in an area that is free of PCR-amplified product. Similarly, oligonucleotides used for amplification should be synthesized and purified in an environment free of PCR product.

Modified Pipettes

Contamination of pipetting devices can result in cross-contamination of samples. To eliminate cross-contamination of samples by pipetting devices, positive-displacement pipettes with disposable tips or disposable tips with filters are recommended.

Careful Laboratory Technique

The following precautions should be taken in all aspects of PCR from sample collection to PCR: (i) change gloves frequently, (ii) uncap tubes carefully to prevent aerosols, (iii) minimize sample handling, and (iv) add nonsample components [mineral oil, deoxynucleoside triphosphates (dNTPs), primers, buffer, and enzyme] to the reaction mixture before addition of sample DNA. Cap each tube after the addition of DNA before proceeding to the next sample.

Selection of Controls

For a positive control, select a sample that amplifies weakly but consistently. The use of strong positives will result in the unnecessary generation of large amounts of amplified DNA sequences. Well-characterized negative controls should also be used. The extreme sensitivity of the PCR process has the potential to amplify a nucleic acid sequence in a sample that is negative by all other criteria. Finally, multiple reagent controls should be included with each amplification. This is because the presence of a small number of molecules of PCR product in the reagents may lead to sporadic positive results. The reagent controls should contain all the necessary components for the PCR process minus the template DNA.

Conclusion

As the AIDS epidemic continues to grow and spread, there will be an increasing need for sensitive and quantitative assays for HIV. Quantitative tests for monitoring the infected cell load and cell-free particulate virus in infected persons will be needed to monitor the clinical status of the patient and to evaluate the efficacy of new antiviral agents and potential vaccines.

The application of PCR technology to AIDS research opens up exciting new possibilities for the sensitive and specific direct detection and quantitation of HIV. In its short existence, PCR has proven valuable for (i) detecting infection in seronegative persons, (ii) quantifying the virus burden in a patient, (iii) typing HIV infections, (iv) measuring virus expression, (v) early diagnosis of perinatal transmission of HIV, and (vi) resolving indeterminate western blots. As a research tool, the PCR technique is also proving useful for studying variant HIVs, distinguishing the important human retroviruses HTLV-I and HTLV-II, and discovering new pathogenic human retroviruses. Further simplification of PCR technology with the addition of sensitive nonisotopic detection systems requiring less than 1 hour for a quantitative readout should guarantee PCR a significant role in the diagnosis of AIDS and HIV infection.

References

1. Harper MH, Marselle LM, Gallo RC, Wong-Staal F. Proc Natl Acad Sci USA 1986;83:772–776.
2. Shaw GM, Hahn BH, Arya SK, Groopman JE, Gallo RC, Wong-Staal, F. Molecular characterization of human T-cell leukemia (lymphotropic) virus type III in the acquired immune deficiency syndrome. Science 1984;226: 1165–1171.
3. Mullis KB, Faloona FA. Specific synthesis of DNA in vitro via a polymerase-catalyzed chain reaction. Meth Enzymol 1987;155:335–350.
4. Saiki RK, Scharf S, Faloona F, Mullis KB, Horn GT, Erlich HA, Arnheim N. Enzymatic amplification of β-globin genomic sequences and restriction site analysis for the diagnosis of sickle cell anemia. Science 1985;230:1350–1354.
5. Saiki RK, Gelfand DH, Stoffel S, Scharf SJ, Higuchi R, Horn GT, Mullis KB, Erlich HA. Primer-directed enzymatic amplification of DNA with a thermostable DNA polymerase. Science 1988;239:487–491.
6. Schochetman G, Ou C-Y, Jones W. Polymerase chain reaction. J Inf Dis 1986;158:1154–1157.
7. Hart C, Spira T, Moore J, Sninsky J, Schochetman G, Lifson A, Galphin J, Ou C-Y. Direct detection of HIV RNA expression in seropositive subjects. Lancet 1988;ii:596–599.
8. Byrne BC, Li JJ, Sninsky J, Poiesz BJ. Detection of HIV-1 RNA sequences by in vitro DNA amplification. Nucleic Acids Res 1988;16:4165.

9. Ou C-Y, Kwok S, Mitchell SW, Mack DH, Sninsky JJ, Feorino P, Warfield D, Schochetman G. DNA amplification for direct detection of HIV-1 in DNA of peripheral blood mononuclear cells. Science 1988;239:295–297.
10. Kwok S, Mack DH, Mullis KB, Poiesz B, Erlich G, Blair D, Friedman-Kien A, Sninsky JJ. Identification of human immunodeficiency virus sequences by using in vitro enzymatic amplification and oligomer cleavage detection. J Virol 1987;61:1690–1694.
11. Kwok S, Mack DH, Sninsky JJ, Erlich GD, Poiesz BJ, Dock NL, Alter HJ, Mildvan D, Grieco MH. Diagnosis of human immunodeficiency virus in seropositive individuals: viral sequences in peripheral blood mononuclear cells. In: Luciw PA, Steimer KS, eds. HIV Detection by Genetic Engineering Methods.
12. Kellogg DE, Kwok S. Detection of human immunodeficiency virus. In: Innis MA, Gelfand DH, Sninsky JJ, White TJ, eds. PCR Protocols. New York: Academic Press, 1989:337–347.
13. Ou C-Y, Schochetman G. Polymerase chain reaction in AIDS research. In: Erlich HA, Gibbs R, Kazazian HH Jr., eds. Current Communications in Molecular Biology, Polymerase Chain Reaction. New York: Cold Spring Harbor Laboratory, 1989:165–170.
14. Meyerhans A, Cheynier R, Albert J, Beth M, Kwok S, Sninsky J, Morfeldt ML Asjo B, Wain-Hobson S. Temporal fluctuations in HIV quasispecies in vivo are not reflected by sequential HIV isolations. Cell 1989;58:901–910.
15. Goodenow M, Huet T, Saurin W, Kwok S, Sninsky J, Wain-Hobson S. HIV-1 isolates are rapidly evolving quasispecies: evidence for viral mixtures and preferred nucleotide substitutions. J Acquir Immune Defic Synd 1989;2: 344–352.
16. Jackson JB, Kwok SY, Sninsky JJ, Hopsicker JS, Hopsicker JS, Sannerud KJ, Rhame FS, Henry K, Simpson M, Balfour HH Jr. Human immunodeficiency virus type 1 detected in all seropositive symptomatic and asymptomatic individuals. J Clin Microbiol 1990;28:16–19.
17. Kellogg DE, Sninsky JJ, Kwok S. Quantitation of HIV-1 proviral DNA relative to cellular DNA by the polymerase chain reaction. Anal Biochem 1990;189:202–208.
18. Ou C-Y, McDonough SH, Cabanas D, Ryder TB, Harper M, Moore J, Schochetman G. Rapid and quantitative detection of enzymatically amplified HIV-1 DNA using chemiluminescent oligonucleotide probes. AIDS Res Hum Retrovir 1990;6:1323–1329.
19. Schnittman SM, Psallidopoulos MC, Lane HC, Thompson L, Baseler M, Massari F, Fox CH, Salzman NP, Fauci AS. The reservoir for HIV-1 in human peripheral blood is a T cell that maintains expression of CD4. Science 1990;245:305–308.
20. Ho DD, Moudgil T, Alam M. Quantitation of human immunodeficiency virus type 1 in the blood of infected persons. N Engl J Med 1989;321:1625–1626.
21. Coombs RW, Collier AC, Allain J-P, Nikora B, Leuther M, Gjerset GF, Corey L. Plasma viremia in human immunodeficiency virus infection. N Engl J Med 1989;321:1626–1631.
22. Ratner L. Measurement of human immunodeficiency virus load and its relation to disease progression. AIDS Res Hum Retrovir 1989;5:115–119.

23. Lion T, Nighet R, Hutchinson MA, Golomb HM, Brownstein BH. Rapid dot blot quantitation for viral DNA and amplified genes in less than 1,000 cells. DNA 1989;8:361–367.
24. Schnittman SM, Greenhouse JJ, Miltiades BS, Psallidopoulos C, Baseler M, Salzman NP Fauci AS, Lane HC. Increasing viral burden in $CD4^+$ T cells from patients with human immunodeficiency virus (HIV) infection reflects rapidly progressive immunosuppression and clinical disease. Ann Intern Med 1990;113:438–443.
25. Simmonds P, Balfe P, Peutherer JF, Ludlam CA, Bishop JO, Leigh Brown AJ. Human Immunodeficiency virus-infected individuals contain provirus in small numbers of peripheral mononuclear cell and at low copy numbers. J Virol 1990;64:864–872.
26. Spear GT, Ou C-Y, Kessler HA, Moore JL, Schochetman G, Landay AL. Analysis of lymphocytes, monocytes, and neutrophils from human immunodeficiency virus (HIV) infected persons for HIV DNA. J Infect Dis 1990;162: 1239–1244.
27. Hart C, Chang S-Y, Kwok S, Sninsky J, Ou C-Y, Schochetman G. A replication-deficient HIV-1 DNA used for quantitation of the polymerase reaction (PCR). Nucleic Acid Res 1990;18:4029–4030.
28. Clouse KA, Powell D, Washington I, Poll G, Strebel K, Farrar W, Barstad P, Kovacs J, Fauci AS, Folks TM. Monokine regulation of human immunodeficiency virus-1 expression in a chronically infected human T cell clone. J Immunol 1989;142:431–438.
29. Wang AM, Doyle MV, Mark DF. Quantitation of mRNA by the polymerase chain reaction. Proc Natl Acad Sci USA 1989;86:9717–9721.
30. Becker-Andre M, Hahlbrock K. Absolute mRNA quantification using the polymerase chain reaction (PCR). A novel approach by a PCR aided transcript titration assay (PATTY). Nucleic Acid Res 1989;17:9437–9446.
31. Gilliland G, Perrin S, Blanchard K, Bunn HF. Analysis of cytokine mRNA and DNA: detection and quantitation by competitive polymerase chain reaction. Proc Natl Acad Sci USA 1990;87:2725–2729.
32. Murakawa GJ, Zaia JA, Spallone PA, Stephens DA, Kaplan BE, Wallace RB, Rossi JJ. Direct detection of HIV-1 RNA from AIDS and ARC patient samples. DNA 1988;7:287–295.
33. Goudsmit J, Paul DA, Lange J, Speelman H, Noordaa J, Van Der Helm H, deWolf F, Epstein L, Krone W, Wolters E, Loeske J, Coutinho R. Expression of human immunodeficiency virus antigen (HIV-Ag) in serum and cerebrospinal fluid during acute and chronic infection. Lancet 1986;ii:177–180.
34. Kessler H, Blaauw B, Spear J, Paul D, Falk L, Landay A. Diagnosis of human immunodeficiency virus infection in seronegative homosexuals presenting with an acute viral syndrome. JAMA 1987;258:1196–1199.
35. Ranki A, Valle S, Krohn M. Long latency precedes overt seroconversion in sexually transmitted human immunodeficiency virus infection. Lancet 1987; 2:589–593.
36. Simmonds P, Lainson FAL, Cuthbert R, Steel CM, Peutherer JF, Ludlam CA. HIV infection and antibody detection: variable responses to infection in the Edinburgh haemophilic cohort. Br Med J 1987;296:593–598.
37. Ward JW, Schable C, Dickinson GM, Makowka OL, Yanaga GA, Caruana R, Chan H, Salazar F, Schochetman G, Holmberg S. Acute human immuno-

deficiency virus (HIV) infection: antigen detection and seroconversion in immunosuppressed patients. Transplantation 1989;47:722–724.
38. Loche, M, Mach B. Identification of HIV-infected seronegative individuals by a direct diagnostic test based on hybridization to amplified viral DNA. Lancet 1988;ii:418–421.
39. Wolinsky SM, Rinaldo CR, Kwok S, Sninsky JJ, Gupta P, Imagawa D, Farzadegan H, Jacobson LP, Grovit KS, Lee MH, Chmiel JS, Ginzburg H, Kaslow RA, Phair JP. Human immunodeficiency virus type 1 (HIV-1) infection a median of 18 months before a diagnostic western blot: Evidence from a cohort of homosexual men. Ann Intern Med 1989;111:961–972.
40. Hewlett IK, Gregg RA, Hawthorne CA, Mayner RE, Epstein JS, Ou C-Y, Schochetman G, Schumacher RT. Detection of HIV-1 specific DNA and RNA by the polymerase chain reaction prior to seroconversion. *In* Vaccines 89, Modern Approaches to New Vaccines Including Prevention of AIDS, Lerner RA, Ginsberg H, Chanock RM, Brown B, eds. Cold Spring Harbor: Cold Spring Harbor Laboratory, 1989:167–172.
41. Imagawa DT, Lee MH, Wolinsky SM, Sano K, Morales F, Kwok S, Sninsky JJ, Nishanian PG, Giorgi J, Fahey JL, Dudley J, Visscher B, Defels R. Human immunodeficiency virus type 1 infection in homosexual men who remain seronegtive for prolonged periods. N Engl J Med 1989;320:1458–1462.
42. Horsburgh CR Jr, Ou C-Y, Jason J, Holmberg SD, Longini IM, Schable C, Mayer KH, Lifson AR, Schochetman G, Ward JW, Rutherford GW, Evatt BL, Seage GR, Jaffe HW. Duration of human immunodeficiency virus infection before detection of antibody. Lancet 1989;ii:637–640.
43. Jackson JB, MacDonald KL, Cadwell J, Sullivan C, Kline WE, Hanson M, Sannerud KJ, Stramer SL, Fildes NJ, Kwok, SY, Sninsky JJ, Bowman RJ, Polesky HF, Balfour HH, Osterholm MT. Absence of HIV infection in blood donors with indeterminate western blot tests for antibody to HIV-1. N Engl J Med 1990;322:217–220.
44. George JR, Rayfield MA, Phillips S, Heyward WL, Krebs JW, Odehouri K, Soudre R, DeCock K, Schochetman G. Efficacies of U.S. Food and Drug Administration-licensed HIV-1 screening enzyme immunoassays for detecting antibodies to HIV-2. AIDS 1989;4:321–326.
45. Ray F, Salaun D, Lesbordes JL, Gadelle S, Ollivier-Henry F, Barré-Sinoussi F, Chermann J-C, Georges A-J. HIV-1 and HIV-2 double infection in Central African Republic. Lancet 1986;ii:1391–1392.
46. Rey MA, Girard PM, Harzic M, Madjar JJ, Brun-Vezinet F, Saimot AG. HIV-1 and HIV-2 double infection in French homosexual male with AIDS-related complex. Lancet 1987;i:388–389.
47. Foucault C, Lopez O, Jourdan G, Fournel JJ, Perret P, Gluckman JC. Double HIV-1 and HIV-2 seropositivity among blood donors. Lancet 1987; i:165–166.
48. Rayfield M, DeCock K, Heyward WL, Goldstein L, Krebs J, Kwok S, Lee S, McCormick J, Moreau JM, Odehouri K, Schochetman G, Sninsky J, Ou C-Y. Mixed human immunodeficiency virus (HIV) infection of an individual: demonstration of both HIV type 1 and HIV type 2 proviral sequences by polymerase chain reaction. J Infect Dis 1988;158:170–176.
49. Centers for Disease Control. AIDS due to HIV-2 infection—New Jersey. MMWR 1988;37:33–35.

50. Rogers MF, Ou C-Y, Rayfield M, Thomas PA, Schoenbaum EE, Abrams E, Krasinski K, Selwyn PA, Moore J, Kaul A, Grimm KT, Bamji M, Schochetman G, the New York City Collaborative Study of Maternal HIV Transmission and Montefiore Medical Center HIV Perinatal Transmission Study Group. Use of the polymerase chain reaction for early detection of the proviral sequences of human immunodeficiency virus in infants born to seropositive mothers. N Engl J Med 1989;320:1649–1654.
51. Rogers MF, Ou C-Y, Kilbourne B, Schochetman G. Advances and problems in the diagnosis of HIV infection in infants. In Pizzo PA, Wilfert CM, eds. Pediatric AIDS, The Challenge of HIV Infection in Infants, Children and Adolescents. Baltimore: Williams & Wilkins, 1990:159–174.
52. Chadwick EG, Yogev R, Kwok S, Sninsky JJ, Kellogg DE, Wolinsky SM. Enzymatic amplification of the human immunodeficiency virus in peripheral blood mononuclear cells from pediatric patients. J Infect Dis 1989;160:954–959.
53. Pizzo PA, Eddy J, Falloon J, Ballis FM, Murphy RF, Moss H, Wolters P, Brouwers P, Jarosinki P, Rubin M, Broder S, Yarchoan R, Brunetti A, Maha M, Nusinoff-Lehrman S, Poplack DG. Effect of continuous intravenous infusion of zidovudine (AZT) in children with symptomatic HIV infection. N Engl J Med 1988;319:889–896.
54. Larder BA, Darby G, Richman DD. HIV with reduced sensitivity to zidovudine (AZT) isolated during prolonged therapy. Science 1989;246:1731–1734.
55. Larder BA, Kemp SD. Multiple mutations in HIV-1 reverse transcriptase confer high-level resistance to zidovudine (AZT). Science 1989;246:1155–1158.
56. Boucher CAB, Tersmette M, Lange JMA, Kellam P, de Goede REY, Mulder JW, Darby G, Goudsmit J, Larder BA. Zidovudine sensitivity of human immunodeficiency viruses from high-risk, symptom-free individuals during therapy. Lancet 1990;336:585–590.
57. Kwok S, Kellogg DE, McKinney N, Spasic D, Goda L, Levenson C, Sninsky JJ. Effects of primer-template mismatches on the polymerase chain reaction: human immunodeficiency virus type 1 model studies. Nucleic Acids Res 1990;18:999–1005.
58. Higuchi R, Kwok S. Avoiding false positives with PCR. Nature 1989;339: 237–238.
59. Longo MC, Berninger MS, Hartley JL. Use of uracil DNA glycosylase to control carry-over contamination in polymerase chain reactions. Gene 1990; 93:125–128.
60. Sninsky JJ, Gates C, McKinney N, Birch D, Akers J, Lawyer F, Gelfand D. dUTP and uracil-N-glycolase in the polymerase chain reaction: a resolution to carryover (manuscript in preparation).
61. Sheppard HA, Ascher MS, Busch MP, Sohmer PR, Stanley M, Luce MC, Chimera JA, Madej R, Rodgers GC, Lynch C, Kayam-Bashi H, Murphy EE Jr, Eble B, Bradford WZ, Royce RA, Winklestein W Jr. A multicenter proficiency trial of gene amplification (PCR) for the detection of HIV-1.
62. Saiki RK, Bugawan TL, Horn GT, Mullis KB, Erlich HA. Analysis of enzymatically amplified beta-globin and HLA DQ, alpha with allele-specific oligonucleotide probes. Nature 1986;324:163–165.
63. Farzadegan H, Polis MA, Wolinsky SM, Rinaldo CR Jr, Sninsky JJ, Kwok S, Griffith RL, Kaslow RA, Phair JP, Polk BF, Saah AJ. Loss of human

immunodeficiency virus type 1 (HIV-1) antibodies with evidence of viral infection in asymptomatic men. Ann Intern Med 1988;108:785–790.

64. Saiki R, Walsh R, Levenson CH, Erlich HA. Genetic analysis of amplified DNA with immobilized sequence-specific oligonucleotide probes. Proc Natl Acad Sci USA, 1989;86:6230–6234.

8 Human Immunodeficiency Virus Culture

MARK A. RAYFIELD

Although serologic assays are capable of identifying prior exposure to human immunodeficiency virus (HIV), they cannot alone demonstrate whether a person is currently harboring the virus. The first method used to ascertain if a blood specimen contained HIV was cocultivation with stimulated primary human lymphocytes or continuous human T-cell lines and monitoring the culture supernatants for the presence of reverse transcriptase. Although virus isolation has proven to be a poor diagnostic tool because of its relative insensitivity, high costs, and lengthy time requirements, culture has served as the standard by which all other diagnostic tests have been judged and established. Further, virus culture remains the steadfast route by which new variants are identified, isolated, and initially characterized. The emphasis of this chapter is to delineate the impact of a number of related fields of study, including epidemiology, applied serology, classical viral morphology, and molecular virology, on the culture and characterization of HIV specimens. In so doing we point out both the advantages and disadvantages of the current approaches to virus isolation.

Evaluation and Selection of Culture Specimens

It is generally appreciated that the success rate of clinical cultures depends on identification of individuals approprite for culture as well as the timing and method of sampling. In course, each of these elements determines the quality of the specimen and thus the likelihood of success. When screening and selecting candidates on the basis of serologic data, it is important to remember that the positive predictive value (number of true-positive tests/total number of positive tests) of the assay is proportional to the true prevalence of infection within the test population and as such is decreased among low-prevalence populations. For example, the persistence of indeterminate or anomalous serologic findings in an individual at increased risk of HIV infection would warrant further analysis of virologic markers. Conversely, within a low-prevalence population similar findings are not singularly suggestive of HIV infection.[1,2] Further, consideration should be given to questions related to the timing and mode of sampling. In the absence of overt evidence of increased viral replication, the choice should be tissue or fluid likely to contain cells that are actively expressing infectious virus. In perinatal studies, these issues are compounded by reduced sample volumes and difficulties in distinguishing residual maternal immunity from the infant's nascent serologic response. On such occasions, direct detection by amplification methods such as the polymerase chain reaction (PCR) often best serve the immediate diagnostic needs for virologic markers.[3] Frank virus isolation thus is not always necessary for diagnostic purposes, but the choice of detection methods need not be mutually exclusive.

There is a strong correlation between the number of circulating cells carrying proviral DNA copies of HIV, which indicates infectious burden, and the frequency of isolation. In situ hybridization analysis of blood and lymphatic tissues indicates that of the order of only 1 in 10,000 to 1 in 100,000 peripheral blood mononuclear cells (PBMCs) are actively replicating virus.[4] Estimates of the number of PBMCs that might serve as infectious centers have also been derived from limiting dilution culture studies in vitro, using methods that detect active HIV replication such as p24 antigen capture, the reverse transcriptase assay, or RNA specific probing.[5–8] As the virus burden rises from 1 proviral DNA copy in 3,000 PBMCs to 1 in 1,000 or more, the frequency of isolation increases, generally following the rate of progression to CDC stage IV criteria within the patient.[8,9] This is not to say that culture is absolutely linked to disease progression, because successful isolations may result from PBMCs of asymptomatic, CDC stage II persons.[10] The critical measure remains the number of cells carrying HIV proviral DNA copies that are replicating or that can be induced to replicate HIV as infectious centers in the culture inoculum. The cumulative findings from these studies indicate that not only does the number of HIV-infected PBMCs increase during disease progression, but the percentage of these cells actively producing virus also rises sharply. These results provide a graphic explaination for the strong correlation between virus isolation rates and prognostic indicators of the clinical disease stages of AIDS.

Culture and Virus Isolation

Reported rates of virus isolation from the blood of HIV-1 antibody-positive persons range from 65% to 100%.[11,12] HIV has also been occasionally isolated from lymphoid tissues, plasma, saliva, semen, tears, brain tissue, cerebral spinal fluid, breast milk, and urine.[13–17] Although HIV has been documented in saliva, tears, and urine, these findings are rare and there is no epidemiologic evidence that contact with these secretions has resulted in infection. The more frequent recovery of HIV from the cerehospinal fluid (CSF) of AIDS patients with neurologic disorders suggested a causal role.[18] Further, the detection of viral antigens or isolation of HIV from plasma before complete seroconversion was initially the only means of demonstrating infection before the development of PCR technology. Therefore, while there are occasions when it may be valuable to attempt isolation from such fluids, the high isolation rates from PBMCs promote the use of whole blood as the principal source of diagnostic material.

Blood should be collected in the presence of an anticoagulant, usually heparin, sodium citrate, or EDTA, then stored at room temperature until the cells are separated. An effort should be made to collect 10–20 ml of blood from adults and 2–5 ml from infants or small children. A partially purfied PBMC preparation, enriched for lymphocytes and adherent mononuclear cells, may be obtained by a single centrifugation through Ficol-Hypaque or similar gradient for lymphocyte separation. The resulting mixed population of cells is ideal for cocultivation and virus isolation. Theoretically, it is best to culture the cells within a few hours of collection but in practice there is little loss of infectivity in unseparated blood held as long as 24 hours before processing. If virus cultivation is to be delayed longer than 24 hours, the PBMCs should be separated and the cells frozen. Cryogenic procedures that yield greater than 80% viability result in minimal loss of infectivity, and HIV may be isolated from specimens properly stored in this manner for longer than 5 years.

Protocols for the isolation of HIV by coculture with primary PBMCs generally require mitogen-stimulated normal donor cells as targets, cultivated at a concentration of 2×10^6 cells/ml. Donor PBMCs are separated by centrifugation over a Ficoll gradient, then precultured at 37°C for 72 hours in RPMI 1640 (GIBCO) media supplemented with 20 m*M* L-glutamine, 20% heat-inactivated fetal calf serum, 5 μg/ml phytohemagglutinin (PHA), and antibiotics as needed. After activation the PHA is removed, and media supplemented with 100–200 U/ml antihuman interferon and 150 U/ml interleukin-2 is added to the culture. PBMCs from the diagnostic specimen are added at an inoculum of 10^6–10^7 cells and the culture supplemented with fresh stimulated normal donor PBMCs at 3-day intervals. Optimal specimen-to-target-cell ratios range from 1:1 to 3:1. Given these cell concentrations, comparable isolation rates may be obtained in culture volumes of 2–20 ml. Isolation rates may vary in culture volumes of less than 2 ml because of the reduced sample size. Material withdrawn at the time of feeding is usually analyzed by the p24 antigen capture assay, reverse transcriptase assay, or PCR for the presence of HIV. Repeatedly positive cultures with a rising titer in quantitative assays are considered indicative of infection. Cultures that remain negative are maintained and monitored for at least 4 weeks (Figure 8.1).

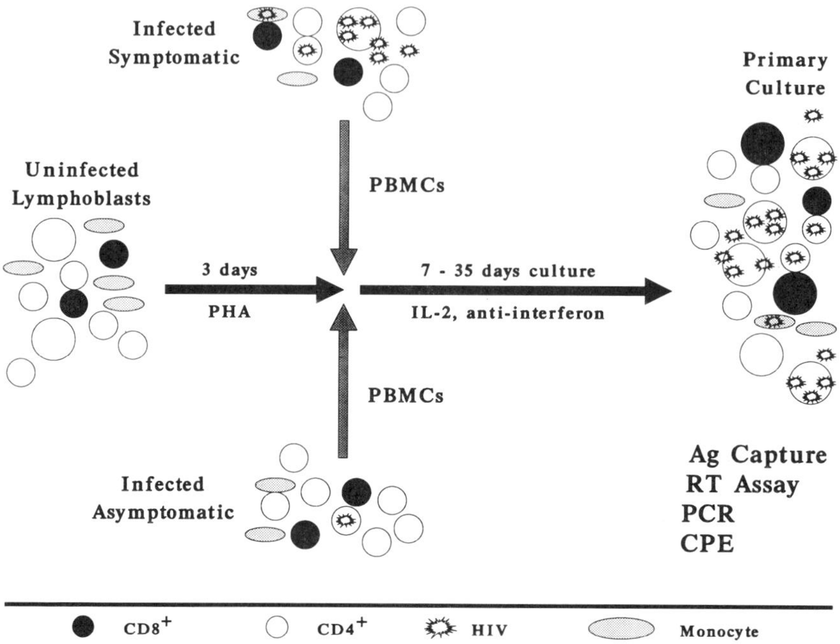

FIGURE 8.1. HIV Isolation protocol. Peripheral blood mononuclear cells (PBMCs) from uninfected donors are pretreated with phytohemagglutin (PHA) to enrich for activated lymphoblasts, which serve as target cells for HIV isolation. Fresh PBMCs from asymptomatic or symptomatic HIV-infected persons are added at specimen to-target-cell ratio >1:1. Resulting mixed-lymphocyte cocultures are monitored regularly for evidence of HIV replication. Abbreviations: Ag capture, antigen capture; CPE, cytopathic effect; PCR, polymerase chain reaction; PBMC, periphiral blond mononuclear cells.

These mixed cultures of immunocompetent cells promote the presentation of a variety of stimuli, including viral antigens as well as heterologous HLA and cell-surface markers that in turn trigger a complex cascade of immune modulators from the participating cells. Among these are the activation of the CD8 suppressor lymphocytes and potential downregulation of CD4 lymphocyte activity. In patients with elevated levels of suppressor-cytotoxic (CD8) T lymphocytes and a low frequency of HIV-expressing cells in circulation, suppression in vitro may be sufficient to inhibit isolation. To avoid these difficulties two approaches are being developed; direct stimulation of selected T-cell populations in mixed lymphocyte cultures[19] and, alternatively, the targeted culturing of only CD4 lymphocytes in the absence of CD8 cells.[20] Although culture methods that exclusively target CD4 lymphocytes have the disadvantage of loss of potentially productive synergy between heterologous cell types, cell-sorting studies indicate that the preponderance of virus in the peripheral blood system is harbored in the CD4 lymphocyte subset.[21,22]

The initial propagation of HIV was achieved in neoplastic T-cell lines, and much of the large-scale preparation of virus continues to be done in continuous lymphoid cell lines.[23,24] Most such cell lines in use today are subclones of previously established lines that have been selected for favorable growth of HIV. Continuous cell lines have the advantages of consistency, availability, and lower maintenance costs over primary donor PBMC cultures. Derivations of the cutaneous human T-cell lymphoma lines HUT-102 and HUT-78, including H9, are widely used. Cell lines that were derived from acute lymphoblastic leukemias include MT2, MT4, MOLT-3, MOLT-4, and CEM. These lines vary in their surface expression of CD4, and certain subclones, especially derivatives of CEM, are noted for their elevated expression of CD4 resulting in heightened HIV susceptibility. The H9, MOLT-3, MT4, and CEM cell lines are most frequently used in initial isolations although they lack the sensitivity of primary PBMC cultures. Although these continuous lines are maintained as suspension cultures, the MT4 cell line and the CEM.SS derivative line of CEM have the advantage of adherence to poly-L lysine-coated plastics, which is useful in quantal assays.[25] Finally, the human myeloid cell line U937 has proven useful in studies of host cell tropisms of HIV isolates because it expresses many of the characteristics of mature tissue macrophages. Studies suggest that isolates derived from monocytic cell lines or primary macrophage/monocyte cultures will infect both monocytic and lymphocytic lines, while those isolated in lymphoblasts are restricted to lymphocytic lines.[26]

Detection and Characterization

A number of methodologies are available for the detection of HIV replication in vitro, including immunoadsorbance assays, electron microscopy, nucleic acid probes, and viral-specific enzymatic assays. Reverse transcriptase and antigen capture assays can provide direct quantification of HIV in culture; when applied to infectious center studies in vitro they allow estimates of virus burden in the host. Limiting dilution analysis of syncytial formation and resulting CPE is useful in conjunction with neutralizing antisera to serotype isolates. Of these, the HIV-1 p24-based antigen capture assay is today the most widely used method of monitoring diagnostic cultures.

Reverse Transcriptase Assay

The usual methods for measuring reverse transcriptase activity in culture are recent modifications of earlier methods for analyzing this distinctive enzyme of retroviruses.[27] Briefly, virus is pelleted by differential centrifugation from the supernatants of cocultures and solubilized in the presence of a mild detergent. The viral lysate serves as a source of reverse transcriptase, which is detected by the incorporation of labeled nucleotides into acid-insoluble nucleic acid in the presence of Mg^{2+} and an RNA template primer. Duplicate samples are assayed per culture, and acid-insoluble label is collected on a filter then measured in a beta scintillation counter or following autoradiography. In general, specimens with threefold increases over the values observed in negative control cultures are considered reactive, and rising titers should be repeatedly observed over a 3- to 6-day interval to confirm a positive culture. This also serves as a quantitation of reverse transcriptase activity and is proportional to the original concentration of HIV in the coculture. Obviously, analysis of HIV growth rates in culture depend on comparable reverse transcriptase activity between isolates, and isolates with nonlethal mutations in the *pol* gene could be quite distinct in their growth patterns.[28] Modifications to this technique include adaptation to a 96-well microtiter format, the use of semiautomatic cell harvesters, and autoradiographic quantitation methods.[29]

This assay is excellent for the detection of retroviruses, but it lacks specificity for HIV and requires 7–10 days of cocultivation before detectable levels of RT activity are observed with most specimens. Although isolation of HTLV-I and HTLV-II has been reported from AIDS patients,[30,31] the frequency of transformation events leading to the successful propagation of these lymphoprolific viruses often requires cultivation periods of more than 4 weeks. Because these viruses also replicate via a reverse transcriptase, consideration should be given for them during the cultivation of specimens for extended periods. Finally, the spurious cocultivation of agents such as the human herpesvirus type-6 group (HHV-6) that infect T lymphocytes will also competitively suppress HIV replication in vitro and inhibit any detection method which relies on active virus production.[32]

Viral Antigen

The methodology of the enzyme-linked immunoassay-based capture and detection of HIV p24 antigen is extensively discussed elsewhere in Chapter 5. This protocol is readily applicable to monitoring supernatants of infected cultures because it permits specific spectrometric quantitation of uncomplexed HIV core antigens. It has the further advantages of low costs, greater sensitivity thus requiring less specimen volume, and greater specificity than the reverse transcriptase (RT) assay.[33] Although commercially available antigen capture assays have a sensitivity sufficient to detect 10–30 pg/ml, most laboratories consider the presence of 30 pg/ml or more indicative of a productive culture. Given a threshold reactivity of 30 pg/ml, repeatedly reactive specimens should show a minimal rise of 100 pg/ml in culture. In a direct comparison of RT activity versus antigen detection for monitoring cultured serial dilutions of HIV-1, the antigen capture method was found to be 100 fold more sensitive in detecting viral replication.[34] Because this assay incorporates antisera to HIV-1, it is highly specific and will not detect other human lymphotrophic viruses such as HTLV-I or HTLV-II. Unfortunately, the sensitivity of current HIV-1-derived assays is to some extent strain specific and is reduced against HIV-2 or distant variants from the prototype HIV-1, which express core antigens with altered epitopes or determinants.

Nucleic Acid Probe

Advances in nucleic acid hybridization technology have provided a number of methods of importance in detecting HIV replication. Principal among these are in situ hybridization, RNA dot blot analysis, and the more recent PCR for amplification of proviral DNA. Most hybridization assays using labeled nucleic acid probes can detect approximately 10 pg of targeted DNA or roughly one proviral DNA copy per 200 cells. Thus the sensitivity of Southern or dot blot hybridizations falls below that needed for direct detection of HIV in the peripheral blood and lymphatic tissues.[35] As noted previously, PCR is the method of choice for direct analysis of infected tissues because of the high degree of amplification it affords. Conversely, each of these approaches is useful in monitoring HIV replication in cocultures. Southern blot analysis can be used to fingerprint the endonuclease cleavage patterns of new isolates; in situ hybridization is useful in identifying specific cells replicating HIV; and dot blot analysis can be used to screen for specific RNA transcripts. PCR often provides the greatest versatility in association with culture. Not all variants within a given isolation attempt will propagate equally well in culture. PCR provides a means of analyzing minor species that will be operationally lost to study as the more agressive variants expand in vitro. To profit from such an approach, the PCR analysis must be initated at the onset of culture or in conjunction with limiting dilution studies. PCR may also be used in a manner analogous to serotyping to genotypically characterize variants within a culture or in conjunction with linker sequences to provide a rapid means of cloning and expressing the genomes of selected isolates.

Cytopathic Effects and Syncytia Formation

As can be inferred from the foregoing, most primary HIV isolates exhibit a higher degree of replication and cytopathology in fresh PBMCs. However, because cytopathic effects (CPE) and syncytia formation are both host cell and isolate dependent, comparative studies are frequently done in continuous cell lines that provide a stable background.[36] Given a stable culture environment the rate of cell death, cytolysis, and fusion may vary greatly between primary isolates. Cell death may follow a general slowing of the mitotic cycle or be independent of cell division, and RT activity need not directly correlate with the extent of CPE present in the culture system.[28] Susceptibility to syncitial formation is also donor dependent in primary PBMCs, and as with the continuous lines most infected cells will die before inclusion in giant cells.[37] For each of these reasons, assays that rely on the quantitation of infectious HIV are best done with isolates after establishment in a continuous cell line.

Microscopic Analysis

Initially used to demonstrate the presence of virus in diagnostic cultures, electron microscopy (EM) is generally supportive in nature and is best suited for morphogenesis studies. Studies of HIV-1 in vitro replication first revealed many features in common with equine infectious anemia and Maedi/Visna viruses of the Lentivirinae.[24] Now recognized as a member of the Lentivirus subfamily, the nascent HIV-1 virion resembles a type C retrovirus particle during the early stages of budding from the plasma membrane. However, the mature enveloped virus has a distinctive electron-dense nucleoid that is condensed into an eccentric, often bar-shaped structure that does not appear to contact the viral envelope.[38] Although its unique structure gives the HIV virion a readily identifiable character, significant viral replication must occur in the culture for EM analysis to be practical.

Indirect immunofluorescence and similar enzyme-linked immunoassays are commonly used in conjunction with standardized antisera to detect HIV replication and define the subcellular loci of replicating viral elements. Culture samples are evaluated and quantified on the basis of the percentage of labeled cells, intensity of the staining, and the labeling pattern. Consequently, these techniques are frequently used to evaluate expansion of the initial isolate or determine the percentage of productive cells in large scale culture systems. Cultures are best done in continuous cell lines such as H9, HUT-78, or CEM cells so that the pooled sera or plasma might be standardized and preabsorbed to uninfected cells, thus eliminating nonviral-specific binding. The indirect immunofluorescence assay (IFA) and comparable immunoenzyme assays have the advantages of ease of use, specificity and sensitivity, especially with respect to the cell-associated glycoproteins of the viral envelope.[39] The principal disadvantage of the microscopic immunoassays is that they are highly subjective, yet such methods provide a practical alternative to the radio immunoprecipitation assay (RIPA) in detection of the glycosylated HIV envelope proteins.

Western Blot and RIPA

RIPA and western blot technology, in conjunction with well-characterized sera, can be used to fingerprint the protein banding patterns of new viral isolates by polyacrylamide gel electrophoresis (PAGE). These assays are not quantitative, but the observed banding pattern is characteristic of the cultured isolate[40] and may be used to distinguish HIV variants. As is the case with their respective diagnostic applications, protocols for partial purification, reduction, and generation of the PAGE product have not been standardized and may vary greatly among laboratories. Thus the reported migration patterns for a given isolate may differ; this is especially true for the apparent molecular weights for glycosylated viral proteins. Distinctions are also noted in the expression and maturation of HIV proteins in differing continuous cell lines or host cells.

Summary

In conclusion, although advances in serologic and biochemical detection techniques have largely surplanted virus culture as efficient diagnostic tools, related advances continue to be made in HIV isolation that extend its role as a prognostic standard. It is because of the strong correlation between isolation rates and circulating virus burden that culture remains a relevant marker in monitoring disease progression and theraputic intervention. Regardless of its costs and stringent specimen requirements, culture will thus continue to serve the unique need for providing a definable infectious entity to the researcher for study.

References

1. Jackson JB, MacDonald KL, Cadwell J, Sullivan C, Kline WE, Hanson M, et al. Absence of HIV infection in blood donors with indeterminate western blot tests for antibody to HIV-1. N Engl J Med 1990;25:217–222.
2. Dock NL, Kleinman SH, Rayfield MA, Schable CA, Williams AE, Dodd RY. Status of human immunodeficiency virus infection in individuals with persistently indeterminate western blot patterns: prospective studies in a low prevalence population. Arch Int Med 1991;151:525–530.
3. Rogers M, Ou CY, Rayfield MA, Thomas PA, Schoenbaum EE, Abrams E, et al. Polymerase chain reaction for early detection of HIV proviral sequences in infants born to HIV-seropositive mothers. N Engl J Med 1989;320(25): 1649–1654.
4. Harper ME, Marselle LM, Gallo RC, Wang-Staal F. Detection of lymphocytes expressing human T-lymphotropic virus type III in lymph nodes and peripheral blood from infected individuals by in situ hybridization. Proc Natl Acad Sci USA 1986;83:772–776.
5. Richman DD, McCutchan JA, Spector SA. Detecting human immunodeficiency virus RNA in peripheral blood mononuclear cells by nucleic acid hybridization. J Infect Dis 1987;156:823–828.
6. Ulrich PP, Busch MP, El-Beik T, Shiota J, Vennari J, Shiver K, Vyas GN. Assessment of human immunodeficiency virus expression in co-cultures of

peripheral blood mononuclear cells from healthy seropositive subjects. J Med Virol 1988;25:1–10.
7. Ho DD, Moudgil T, Alam M. Quantitation of human immundeficiency virus type 1 in the blood of infected persons. N Engl J Med 321:1625–1626.
8. Simmonds P, Balfe P, Peutherer JF, Ludlam CA, Bishop JO, Leigh Brown AJ. Human immunodeficiency virus-infected individuals contain provirus in small numbers of peripheral mononuclear cells and at low copy numbers. J Virol 1990;64:864–872.
9. Schnittman SM, Greenhouse JJ, Mitiades BS, Psallidopoulos C, Baseler M, Salzman NP, et al. Increasing viral burden in CD4$^+$ T cells from patients with human immunodeficiency virus (HIV) infection reflects rapidly progressive immunosuppression and clinical disease. Ann Intern Med 1990;113:438–443.
10. Jackson JB, Kwok SY, Sninsky JJ, Hopsicker JS, Sannerud HH, Rhame FS, et al. Human immunodeficiency virus type 1 detected in all seropositive symptomatic and asymptomatic individuals. J Clin Microbiol 28:16–19.
11. Francis DP, Jaffe HW, Fultz PN, Getchell JP, McDougal JS, Feorino PM. The natural history of infection with the lymphadenopathy associated human T lymphocytic virus type III. Ann Intern Med. 1985;103:719–722.
12. Jackson JB. Human immunodeficiency virus type 1 antigen and culture assays. Arch Pathol Lab Med 1990;114:249–254.
13. Levy J, Kaminsky L, Morrow W, Steimer K, Luciw P, Dina D, Hoxie J, Oshiro L. Infection by the retrovirus associated with AIDS. Ann Intern Med 1985;103:694–699.
14. Gaines H, Albert J, Von Sydow M, Sonnerborg A, Chiodi F, Ehrnst A, Strannegard O, Asjo B. HIV antigenemia and virus isolation from plasma during primary HIV infection. Lancet 1987:i:1317–1318.
15. Ho D, Schooley R, Rota R, Kaplan J, Flynn T. HTLV-III in the semen and blood of a healthy homosexual man. Science 1984;226:451–453.
16. Ho D, Rota R, Schooley R, Kaplan J, Allan J, Groopman J, Resnick L, Felsenstein D, Andrews C, Hirsch M. Isolation of HTLV-III from cerebrospinal fluid and neural tissues of patients with neurologic syndromes related to the acquired immundeficiency syndrome. N Engl J Med 1985;313: 1493–1497.
17. Ho D, Byington R, Schooley R, Flynn T, Rota T, Hirsch M. Isolation of HTLV-III from 83 saliva and 50 blood samples from 71 serpositive homosexual men. N Engl J Med 1985;313:1606.
18. Koenig S, Gengelman HE, Orenstein JM, Dal Canto MC, Pezeshkpour GH, Yungbluth M, Janotta F, Aksamit A, Martin MA, Fauci AS. Detection of AIDS virus macrophages in brain tissue from AIDS patients with encephalopathy. Science 1986;233:1089–1093.
19. Walker C, Bettens F, Pichler WJ. Activation of T cells by cross-linking an anti-CD3 antibody with a second anti-T cell antibody: mechanism and subset-specific activation. Eur J Immunol 1987;17:873–880.
20. Walker CM, Moody DJ, Stites DP, Levy JA. CD8$^+$ lymphocytes can control HIV infection in vitro by suppressing virus replication. Science 1986;234: 1563–1566.
21. Schnittman SM, Psallidopoulos MC, Lane HC, Thompson L, Baseler M, Massari F, et al. The reservoir for HIV-1 in human peripheral blood is a T cell that maintains expression of CD4. Science 1990;245:305–308.

22. Spear GT, Ou CY, Kessler HA, Moore JL, Schochetman G, Landay AL. Analysis of lymphocytes, monocytes, and neutrophils from human immunodeficiency virus (HIV) infected persons for HIV DNA. J Infect Dis 1990;162: 1239–1244.
23. Barr-Sinoussi F, Chermann JC, Rey F, Nugeyne MT, Chamaret S, Gruest J, et al. Isolation of a T-lymphotropic retrovirus from a patient at risk for acquired immune deficiency syndrome (AIDS). Science 1983;220:868–871.
24. Popovic M, Sarngadharan MG, Read E, Gallo RC. Detection. isolation and continuous production of cytopathic retroviruses (HTLV-III) from patients with AIDS and pre-AIDS. Science 1984;224:497–500.
25. Tateno M, Levy JA. MT-4 plaque formation can distinguish cytopathic subtypes of the human immunodeficiency virus (HIV). Virology 1988;167: 299–301.
26. Gendelman HE, Baca LM, Husayni H, Turpin JA, Skillman D, Kalter DC, Orenstein JM, Hoover DL, Meltzer MS. Macrophage-HIV interaction: viral isolation and target cell tropism. AIDS 1990;4:221–228.
27. Robert MS, Smith RG, Gallo RC, Sarin PS, Absell JW. Viral and cellular DNA polymerases: comparison of activities on synthetic and natural RNA templates. Science 1972;176:798–800.
28. Cloyd M, Moore B. Spectrum of biological properties of human immunodeficiency virus (HIV-1) isolates. Virology 1990;174:103–116.
29. Spira TJ, Bozeman LH, Holman RC, Warfield DT, Philips SK, Feorino PM. Micromethod for assaying reverse transcriptase. J Clin Microbiol 1987;25: 97–99.
30. Hahn B, Popovic M, Kalyanaraman V, Shaw G, LaMonico A, Weiss S, Wong-Staal F, Gallo R. Detection and characterization of HTLV-II provirus in patients with AIDS. In Gottlieb MS, Groopman JE, eds. Acquired Immune Deficiency Syndrome. New York: Alan R. Liss.
31. Chorta T, Brynes R, Kalyanaraman V, Telfer M, Ramsey R, Mawle A, Palmer E, Feorino P, Evatt B. Transformed T-lymphocytes infected by a novel isolate of human T-cell leukemia virus type II. Blood 1985;66: 1336–1342.
32. Lopez C, Pellet P, Stewart J, Sanderlin K, Black J, Warfield D, Feorino PM. Characteristics of human herpesvirus-6. J Infect Dis 1988;157:1271–1273.
33. Jackson JB, Sannerud K, Rhame FS, Balfour HH. Evaluation of two commercial tests for human immunodeficiency virus antigens in culture supernatant fluid. Am J Clin Pathol 1988;89:788–790.
34. Feorino PM, Forrester B, Warfield DT, Schochetman G. Comparison of antigen assay and reverse transcriptase assay for detecting human immunodeficiency virus in culture. J Clin Microbiol 1987;25:2344–2346.
35. Shaw GM, Hahn BH, Arya SK, Groopman JE, Gallo RC, Wong-Staal F. Molecular characterization of human T-cell leukemia (lymphotropic) virus type III in the acquired immune deficiency syndrome. Science 1984;226: 1165–1171.
36. World Health Organization Global Programme on AIDS. Report of a WHO workshop on the measurement and significance of neutralizing antibody to HIV and SIV. AIDS 1990;4:269–275.

37. Somasundaran M, Robinson HL. A major mechanism of human immundeficiency virus-induced cell killing does not involve cell fusion. J Virol 1987;61:3114–3119.
38. Palmer E, Sporborg C, Harrison A, Martin ML, Feorino P. Morphology and Immunoelectron microscopy of the AIDS virus. Arch. Virol. 1985;85: 189–196.
39. Sandstrom EG, Schooley RT, Ho DD, Byington R, Sarngadharan MG. Detection of human anti-HTLV-III antibodies by indirect immunofluorescence using fixed cells. Transfusion 1985;25:302–312.

9
Use of Flow Cytometry to Monitor HIV Disease

ALAN L. LANDAY and BETSY M. OHLSSON-WILHELM

Lymphocyte subset enumeration using monoclonal antibodies and flow cytometry is a powerful tool in the clinical immunology laboratory. The immunophenotypic profile (i.e., the number of different types of lymphocytes determined by flow cytometry) is used together with in vitro assessments of lymphocyte function and clinical observations to diagnose disease and to predict outcome. In general, the level of different lymphocyte subsets in the peripheral blood is an accurate reflection of the overall immune status of an individual. Immunophenotyping is most commonly used to evaluate immunodeficiencies [i.e., human immunodeficiency virus (HIV) infection] discriminate subtypes of leukemias and lymphomas and in monitoring immune suppression (e.g., OKT3 therapy) and immune reconstitution (e.g., post bone marrow transplant).

Principles of Flow Cytometry

Flow cytometry allows for the correlated multiparametric analysis of large numbers of single cells in suspension.[1–3] Cell suspensions are injected through a nozzle into a flowing sheath fluid that hydrodynamically focuses the cells into the center of the stream in columnar flow. Cells pass single file through a focused light beam, usually generated from either a laser or a mercury arc lamp. Each cell traversing the beam scatters light and emits fluorescence if labeled with a fluorescent reagent. Optical signals (scattered light and fluorescence) are collected through specific filters and photodetectors (photodiodes and photomultiplier tubes). The resultant analog signals are digitized and sent to a computer for processing (Figure 9.1).

Current methodology employs a flow cytometer able to collect two light-scatter parameters (forward/low-angle scatter and 90°/side scatter) and two fluorescence signals (fluorescein and phycoerythrin). Light-scatter signals provide information about cell size as well as cytoplasmic and nuclear characteristics. Fluorescence signals are usually generated from reagents directed at specific cell-surface antigens (markers) and can be

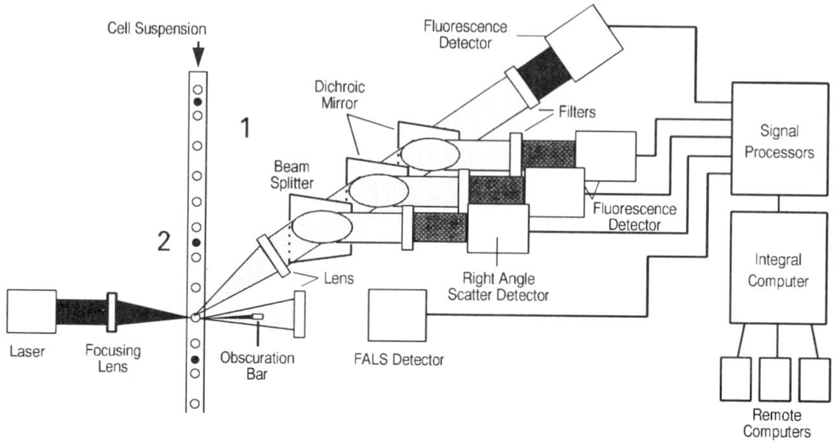

FIGURE 9.1. Schematic representation of modern flow cytometer suitable for clinical work. Stained cells enter flow chamber (1) and pass into center of stream of sheath fluid in single file (2). They are then struck by focused laser beam and emit scattered and fluorescent light, separated according to wavelength by appropriate mirrors and filters. An obscuration bar protects forward-angle light-scatter (FALS) detector from exposure to direct laser beam. Three fluorescence detectors are shown plus detector to measure laser light scattered perpendicular to laser beam by cells. Signals from detectors pass to amplifying processors and then to integral (onboard) computer, which digitizes, stores, and displays the signals. Detailed analysis of data is often most efficient with stand-alone computers.

used to characterize cell subsets as well as the state of activation or differentiation of the cells.

Applications of Flow Cytometry in Monitoring HIV Disease

Methods for Immunophenotyping

Sample Collection

Performing immunophenotypic analysis by flow cytometry begins with attention to sample preparation and staining and with instrument calibration as well as methods for sample and data analysis. In fact, quality assurance for immunophenotypic analysis actually begins at the time of specimen collection. Patient medication should be noted because several commonly used drugs affect light-scatter patterns and cellular autofluorescence. The date and time at which a sample is drawn will affect absolute lymphocyte count (diurnal variation) and should be clearly noted on the requisition slip.[4] If the specimen is to be processed within 6 hours, the recommended anticoagulant is a disodium salt of ethylenediamine-tetraacetic acid (EDTA). This anticoagulant is recommended because laboratory data are usually reported as absolute counts rather than percentages, and it is desirable to perform the white count, differential, and cell marker analysis on the same sample to reduce variability. Six hours is chosen as a maximum because after this time automated white cell counters will begin to reject samples. Recent studies suggest that phenotypic analysis using EDTA as an anticoagulant gives satisfactory results for up to 24 hours.[5] If the specimen will not be processed within 6 hours of collection, heparin or acid citrate dextrose (ACD) may be used as the anticoagulant.[6]

Samples should be transported immediately to the laboratory and stored at 22°C until processed. Transport and storage at 22°C is preferable to 4°C because whole blood samples stored at 4°C frequently demonstrate a significant loss of T-helper cells.[7] More recent data, however, suggest the samples held at 4°C overnight show no appreciable loss of CD4 cells when processed by a whole blood lysis technique.[8] In preparing a sample for staining, the goal is to maintain all cellular components as they were in vivo. For peripheral blood lymphocytes, this means that ideally all lymphocyte subpopulations are preserved while other components that may interfere with the identification of lymphocytes during the analysis phase are eliminated. Thus, whole blood lysis is the recommended method for sample preparation. Because all types of leukocytes will be present in a lysed whole blood preparation, gating by light-scatter properties is then used during analysis to exclude monocytes, granulocytes, and erythrocyte ghosts from consideration.

Choice of Immunophenotyping Panel

In clinical medicine, a complete immunophenotypic profile includes enumeration of several lymphocyte subsets.[9] Many of the monoclonal antibodies used for lymphocyte subset enumeration react with important functional structures on the cell surface for example, anti-CD3 antibodies reacts with the T-cell receptor for antigen (Table 9.1). Those antibodies with similar reactivity, that is, those which react with the same cell-surface molecule, are clustered for naming purposes and have been given the designations CD1 through CD78; the CD in these names stands for cluster differentiation. Specific immunophenotyping information reported on patients should include both the cluster designation examined and the particular monoclonal antibody utilized, for example, CD4 (OKT4A), CD3 (T3), or CD8 (Leu2a).[10,11]

A typical two-color immunofluorescence staining panel with the lymphocyte subsets defined is provided in Table 9.2. Fluorescein and phycoerythrin are the two fluorochromes recommended, and all antibodies are directly labeled. Two-color as opposed to single-color immuno-

TABLE 9.1. Functional role for cell surface antigens (adhesion molecules, enzymes, growth factor receptors).

Cluster differentiation	Ligand	Cellular distribution
CD2	CD58 receptor	T cell, NK subset
CD3	T-cell antigen–receptor complex	T cells
CD4	Class II MHC/HIV receptor	T-cell subsets, monocytes
CD8	Class I MHC	T and NK subset
CD10	Neutral endopeptidase	Pre B cells, PMN
CD11a	LFA-1	Leukocytes
CD11b	CR3, cell adhesion molecule	Mono/myeloid, NK, T cell subset
CD11c	CR4, cell adhesion molecule	Mono/myeloid, NK, T cell subset
CD13	Amino endopeptidase	Monocyte, PMN
CD15	X hapten	PMN, activated T subset
CD16	IgG receptor III	NK, PMN, T subset
CD18	Cell adhesion beta subunit	Leukocytes
CD21	Complement receptor-2	B cells
CD23	Fc epsilon receptor	B cells
CD25	IL-2 receptor	T and B subsets, activated T cells
CD26	Dipeptidylpeptidase IV	T subset
CD32	IgG receptor II	Monocyte, PMN, B cells
CD35	CR1	B cells, monocyte, PMN, RBC
CD40	Homology NGF receptor	B cells
CD41a	gp IIb/IIIa	Platelets
CD43	Leucosialin	T cells, PMN
CD44	Pgpl homing receptor	Leukocytes
CD45	Leukocyte common antigen	Leukocytes T and B
CD54	ICAM	Activated BT, macrophages
CD56	N-CAM	NK, T subset
CD57	Myelin-associated glycoprotein	NK, T subset
CD58	LFA 3	Leukocytes
CD64	IgG receptor I	Monocytes, macrophages
CD71	Transferrin receptor	Proliferating cells

TABLE 9.2. Suggested monoclonal antibody (MAb) combinations for routine immunophenotyping.

Monoclonal antibody combination	Purpose
IgG/IgG2[a]	Isotype control
CD45/CD14[b]	Percent lymphocytes in analysis region
CD3/CD4	T-helper/inducer subset
CD3/CD8	T-suppressor/cytotoxic subset
CD3/CD16 + CD56	Total T cells/total NK cells
CD3/CD19	Total B cells

[a] For each combination, first MAb is labeled with fluorescein isothiocyanate and second with phycoerythrin.

[b] This MAb combination can be run first to determine approprite region on light scatter display for lymphocyte population. All other samples from same patient must be run using this region. IgG, immunoglobulin G; NK, natural killer cells.

fluorescence analysis is strongly recommended. Less blood is required (a factor especially important for pediatric specimens), and there are fewer tubes to handle. Further, far more information can be obtained for less cost. Using two-color staining, it is possible to determine whether CD4$^+$ (helper/inducer) and CD8$^+$ (suppressor/cytotoxic) cells are T cells. Monocytes that are CD4$^+$ CD3$^-$ and natural killer (NK) cells which are CD8$^+$ CD3$^-$ can be excluded electronically and thus not counted as they would be using single-color staining. Finally, T cells and NK cells can be enumerated simultaneously to make sure that the T cells that are CD56$^+$ are not included in the NK cell count as well as in the T-cell count (Figure 9.2).

The monoclonal antibodies (MAbs) in the first two samples of Table 9.2 are controls. The immunoglobulin G (IgG) isotype control establishes whether nonspecific binding of IgG-I or IgG-II occurs with each patient's cells, and indicates where to set the integration cursors (boundaries that are set to determine the percentage of positively stained cells).[12] These isotype controls are chosen such that they match the isotypes of the specific antibodies used in the recommended panel. If there is nonspecific

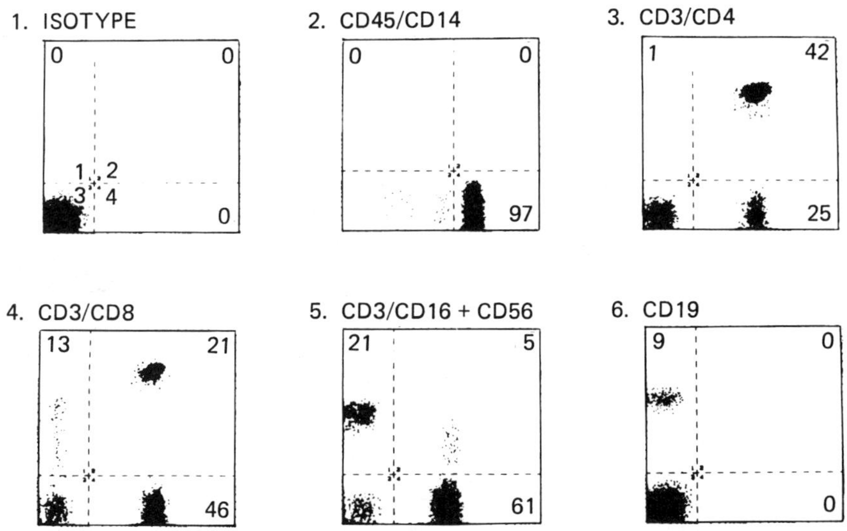

FIGURE 9.2. Dot plots of two-color immunofluorescence staining. Sample number and antibodies correspond to those listed in Table 9.2; the cursors (dotted horizontal and perpendicular lines) are set according to isotype control; in sample 2, however, perpendicular cursor is set to distinguish CD45^{bright} (lymphocytes) and CD45^{dim} (granulocytes). Numbers on histograms give percentage of cells shown in quadrant 1 (PE-stained only), quadrant 2 (dual-stained), and quadrant 4 (FITC only). The unstained cells are in quadrant 3. Increasing FITC staining is toward right along *x* axis and increasing PE staining toward top of each histogram along *y* axis.

binding with the isotype control or with other reagents, 50 μl of neat normal human sera added to the sample tube just before adding the MAbs may reduce the nonspecific binding.

Sample 2 (Table 9.2) should be run first for each patient to determine where the lymphocytes fall on the forward-scatter by right-angle scatter histogram. The CD45 reagent identifies all the leukocytes, while CD14 stains the monocytes. The lymphocytes are differentiated from neutrophils on the basis of their density of CD45 ($CD45^{dim}$ neutrophils/$CD45^{bright}$ lymphocytes). The MAbs in this sample allow the percentage of lymphocytes ($CD45^{bright}/CD14^{-}$) in the gated light-scatter analysis region to be determined.[13] This presumes that the flow cytometry operator has set the lymphocyte analysis region to include all the lymphocytes. The percentage of events in the selected lymphocyte region that are $CD45^{bright}$ $CD14^{-}$ should be between 90% and 100% on all specimens, and blood should be restained if the value is not at least 85%. The percentage of lymphocytes obtained from leukocyte samples should be used to correct the values from the other MAb samples.

Quality Control for Lymphocyte Immunophenotyping

Several checks on immunophenotyping results are used by experienced cytometrists to determine whether flow results are accurate. First, the 'lymphosum' or sum of [T + B + NK] should approach 100% after each of these values is corrected for the "percentage of lymphocytes in the lymphocyte region" as determined from the CD45/CD14 tube (sample 2 of the panel in Table 9.2). This serves as a check on the overall accuracy of the immunophenotyping results. For example, suppose the measured values are T = 70%, B = 10%, and NK = 12%, $CD45^{bright}$ $CD14^{-}$ = 92%; then corrected values are T = 76%, B = 11%, NK = 13%, and lymphosum = 100%. This result is reasonable. If the lymphosum is 85% or 120%, however, the cytometrist should check for clerical errors, cursor setting errors, light-scatter distortions, or staining errors. This variability may also be caused by some underlying biologic process. Either all or select samples from the panel can be restained and rerun to validate or rectify the results. A second useful check is whether the sum of $CD4^{+}$ + $CD8^{+}$ approaches the $CD3^{+}$ cells within ±10% of the $CD3^{+}$ value. In some people this will not be the case for one of two reasons. First, the NK cells express $CD8^{+}$, and if a person has many $CD8^{+}$ NK cells, their $CD4^{+}$ + $CD8^{+}$ values may be greater than the $CD3^{+}$ value by >10%. Second, the presence of the recently described subset of $CD3^{+}$ 4^{-} 8^{-} gamma/delta cells will tend to lower the $CD4^{+}$ + $CD8^{+}$ value, making it less than the CD3 value by >10%. Keeping these two exceptions in mind, checking whether the $CD4^{+}$ + $CD8^{+}$ values and $CD3^{+}$ values are approximately equal in number can prevent many gross errors. Another check is to see that the $CD3^{+}$ values in tubes 3, 4, 5, and 6 are identical.

Flow-cytometric evaluation of the immune system is an extremely valuable technology for prognosis and in assessing the efficacy of therapy for HIV disease. Research is under way to permit evolution of clinical flow cytometry to simplify quality control and guarantee accuracy and reproducibility of results. At present, the best way to be certain that a CD4 value is accurate is to obtain a complete immunophenotypic profile (see Table 9.2) on the individual and use the checks for accuracy of the data suggested above. Recently, a MAb cocktail method has been proposed that allows one to monitor the major lymphocyte subsets in a single sample. This method optimizes accuracy of $CD4^+$ lymphocyte assessment and provides simultaneous enumeration of four other lymphocyte subsets ($CD3^+$ $CD8^+$, $CD3^+$ $CD4^-$ $CD8^-$, $CD19^+$ $CD20^+$, $CD16^+$ $CD56^+$ $CD8^-$; Figure 9.3). This method has the potential for providing accurate $CD4^+$ cell counts on small volumes of blood (100–200 μl), which would be valuable in monitoring pediatric patients with HIV infection. This method requires careful titration of the reagents as well as further development of specialized analytical software to streamline data processing before it will be ready for routine clinical application.[14]

Many of the issues described have been discussed by a national panel of experts. A consensus document (H42-P) for immunophenotypic analysis by flow cytometry has been published by the National Committee for Clinical Laboratory Standards and is available from this organization for laboratory use.[15]

Instrument Quality Control and Standardization

Once stained, the samples are ready for analysis on the flow cytometer. However, instrument performance must first be assessed and qualified to

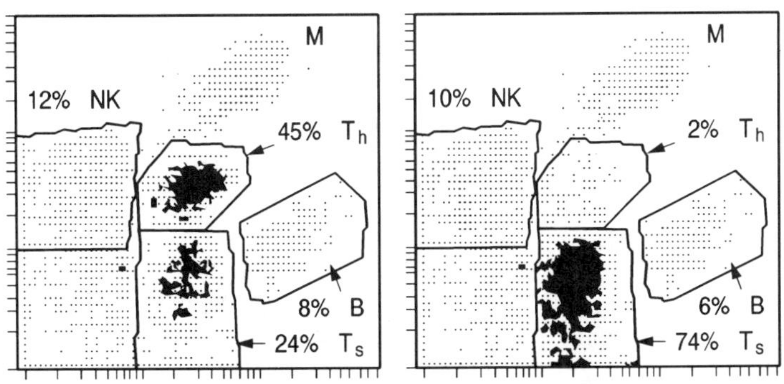

FIGURE 9.3. Cocktail staining: (left) normal healthy individual and (right) AIDS patient (HIV infected). Leukocyte-enriched preparations were stained using monoclonal antibody cocktail.[14] Unlabeled cells in bottom left-hand corner of HIV-infected patient's histogram represent contaminating neutrophils or unlysed red cells. M, monocytes; T_h, $CD3^+$ $CD4^+$; T_s, $CD3^+$ $CD8^+$; B, $CD19^+$ $CD20^+$; NK, $CD16^+$ $CD3^-$; M, $CD14^+$.

ensure that accurate test results will be obtained. Instrument set up typically involves running three different types of materials: (i) uniform particles, (ii) a fluorescence sensitivity control, and (iii) an unstained normal whole-blood sample prepared in parallel with the test samples. Uniform particles provide the easiest check on instrument precision (i.e., reproducibility under a fixed set of instrument conditions) and can be a valuable tool in assessing potential causes if suboptimal performance is observed. The fluorescence sensitivity control consists of stained plastic particles or a stained and fixed biologic material (such as thymocytes). This material allows verification of the instrument's fluorescence sensitivity as demonstrated by the resolution of unstained and dimly stained material. The results obtained by running these quality control materials should also be recorded in a laboratory logbook and graphed daily. A sample of unstained lysed normal whole blood should also be run to verify the total system, including optics, fluidics, and lysing technique. The sensitivity control will also allow standardization of the instrument from day to day so that possible changes in the density of certain antigens, such as CD4, can be accurately documented.

Immune Subset Alterations in HIV Infection

The individual course of disease progression between HIV infection and development of AIDS is highly variable. Flow cytometric evaluation using MAbs against cell surface differentiation antigens provides a powerful tool to assess the extent of immunologic damage and to predict survival in individual patients (Figure 9.4). A classification scheme based on nonrandom development of immunologic abnormalities assessed by

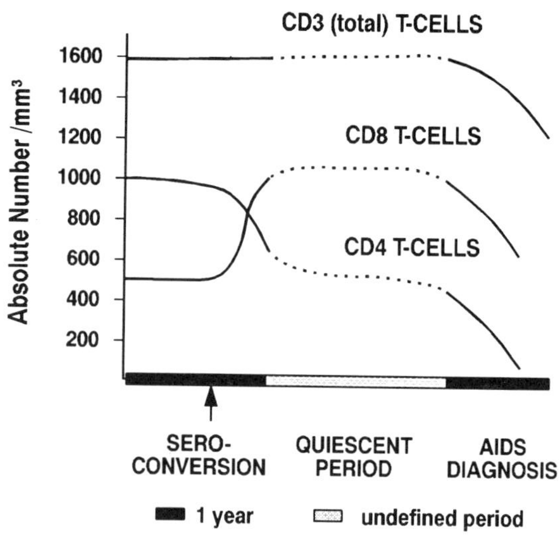

FIGURE 9.4. Pattern of CD4, CD8, and CD3 T-cell changes during HIV disease.

flow cytometry is useful in staging both symptomatic and asymptomatic HIV-infected individuals.[16] In addition, flow-cytometric information can be used to determine whether treatment with antiviral drugs is appropriate or whether it has been effective in arresting immunologic deterioration. As described here, $CD4^+$ cell level and the proportion of $CD8^+$ cells that are $CD38^+$ (marker of activation and immaturity) are the two most informative lymphocyte subset parameters for predicting survival in HIV infection.[17–19] Results from the Multicenter AIDS Cohort Study support monitoring of the $CD4^+$ lymphocyte count at 3- to 6-month intervals during the HIV-seropositive period.[20] For routine monitoring of HIV-infected individuals, the panel of antibodies described in Table 9.2 would be sufficient.

Additional combinations of antibodies may be included ($CD8^+$, $CD38^+$) if of interest to the laboratory. Three-color flow cytometry may be necessary for some antibody combinations because of overlap of subsets. For example, CD8 and CD38 antigens are expressed on T cells and NK cells, and one would require three-color flow cytometry to accurately evaluate the $CD8^+$ and $CD38^+$ T cells. In this case the third dye might be allophycocyanin, which is excited in the red portion of the spectrum. Three-color flow cytometry does require additional controls as well as a second laser, depending on the dye combinations used. Therefore, this technique is still relegated to the research lab and does not yet appear in the routine clinical setting.

$CD4^+$ Cells and Subsets

Four stages of $CD4^+$ cell loss occur during HIV disease.[19] In the first stage, during the first 12 to 18 months after seroconversion, the mean $CD4^+$ cell level falls from $1{,}000/mm^3$ to $600/mm^3$. During the second stage, which can last several years, CD4 levels are relatively stable, although some studies have demonstrated a small but steady fall in $CD4^+$ cell number during the asymptomatic period.[21] Further rapid $CD4^+$ cell loss leads to the development of frank AIDS and characterizes the third stage. In the fourth stage, from AIDS diagnosis to death, $CD4^+$ cell levels fall even further. $CD4^+$ cell decline probably results at least in part from failure to suppress in vivo HIV replication. $CD4^+$ cell levels are highly prognostic for predicting survival, especially during the last two stages, and death occurs within 1 year in about 80% of untreated people whose level has fallen to 10% $CD4^+$ cells/mm^3. $CD4^+$ cell percentages are slightly more predictive for AIDS-free survival than $CD4^+$ cell absolute counts.[22]

Enumeration of functional $CD4^+$ cell subsets with Leu 8, CD29 (4B4 helper/inducer) or CD45RA (Leu18, 2H4, suppressor/inducer) antibodies offers no additional information compared with $CD4^+$ cell measurement alone for evaluating HIV disease progression.[17,18] Although several authors originally suggested that there is preferential early loss of one or another of the $CD4^+$ subsets during a certain stage of HIV disease,[23–25] it is now generally accepted that various functional subpopulations of $CD4^+$ cells defined by these antibodies are lost concurrently.

Other dual-color flow-cytometry studies initiated on $CD4^+$ subsets reveal that AIDS patients have increased numbers of activated $CD4^+$ cells that express CD38 (Leu17) or HLA-DR. These activated cells are not observed in seropositive men without AIDS and may result from or reflect HIV replication in frank AIDS. The observation of activated $CD4^+$ cells was made on AIDS patients who were not on antiretroviral therapy, and studies are now under way to determine whether the proportion of activated $CD4^+$ cells is diminished in individuals on antiretroviral therapy. In other studies, interleukin-2 receptor (CD25) expression, if present, was below detectabe levels, although some investigators have shown a reduction in CD25 expression on cells from HIV-positive individuals.[26]

$CD8^+$ Cells and Subsets

Throughout the course of HIV disease, the total T-cell levels remain fairly constant in spite of the fall in the $CD4^+$ cell number because of the concomitant $CD8^+$ lymphocytosis. A role for homeostatic control of the total T-cell number irrespective of the $CD4^+$ or $CD8^+$ phenotype has been suggested.[20]

About 20% of the $CD8^+$ cells in HIV-seronegative people are $CD38^+$. There is a progressive increase in the proportion of $CD38^+$ (activated and immature) $CD8^+$ cells throughout the course of disease, beginning as soon as there is evidence of HIV infection (seroconversion). In acute Epstein–Barr virus and cytomegalovirus infection, the $CD38^+$ $CD8^+$ cell number also rises quickly during active infection, then diminishes within 1 or 2 months. The decrease occurs at about the time that the herpesvirus infections are cleared by the host. In HIV infection, the $CD38^+$ $CD8^+$ lymphocytosis never abates, and the high $CD38^+$ $CD8^+$ level throughout HIV disease may reflect persistent immune stimulation by HIV. At least some of the $CD38^+$ cells may be anti-HIV T-cytotoxic cells. A high level of $CD38^+$ $CD8^+$ cells, for example, >50%, is an extremely poor prognostic sign in HIV-infected people.

Increases in both $HLA\text{-}DR^+$ and $HLA\text{-}DR^-$ subsets occur in HIV-infected individuals. $HLA\text{-}DR^+$ $CD8^+$ cells are extremely rare in HIV seronegatives (3–8%), and $HLA\text{-}DR^+$ $CD8^+$ cells represent an average of 20–30% of the $CD8^+$ cells in all three HIV-seropositive groups studied. Because the $HLA\text{-}DR^+$ $CD8^+$ proportion was higher in seropositive men than in individuals with AIDS, it is possible that at least some $HLA\text{–}DR^+$ $CD8^+$ cells represent a protective component of the specific anti-HIV immune responses. However, the identification of a high HLA-DR$^+$ CD8$^+$ level as a poor prognostic sign by Stites et al.[27] suggests the alternative hypothesis that the HLA-DR$^+$ CD8$^+$ cells may accelerate the CD4$^+$ cell decline or serve as a marker of HIV activity (Table 9.3).

Total T Cells

The total T-cell level remains relatively stable throughout the period of HIV infection until around the time that AIDS develops. Total leukocyte count, lymphocyte percentage, and absolute lymphocyte number are also relatively stable throughout the pre-AIDS period and are comparable to levels in healthy normal controls. Late in HIV disease, the leukocyte and lymphocyte numbers begin to fall, and lymphopenia and panleukopenia herald the final stages of HIV disease progression. The CD3 percentage remains stable throughout HIV disease and averages approximately 75 ± 10%. In very ill patients who become lymphopenic and leukopenic, the CD3 percentage may be abnormally low, and values of 30–50% are not uncommon. In such patients, most lymphocytes (i.e., up to 80%) are CD8 positive and almost none are CD4 positive.

Gamma/Delta T-Cell-Receptor-Bearing T Cells

The T-cell receptor for antigen is composed of a two-chain molecule that has specificity for antigen and is expressed together with CD3 on the T-cell membrane. The two-chain antigen-specific molecule, or heterodimer,

TABLE 9.3. Immunophenotype profiles in HIV disease.

	Asymptomatic HIV-seropositive homosexual		Late AIDS	
	Percent	Absolute number	Precent	Absolute number
Total leukocytes	—	5800	—	3200
Total lymphocytes	30	1740	25	800
Total T cells	70	1218	72	576
Total B cells	10	174	8	64
Total NK cells	12	209	11	88
CD4$^+$ (T H/I)	30	522	2	16
CD8$^+$ (T S/C)	41	713	70	560
CD4/CD8 ratio	0.73		0.03	
	Proportion of CD8 Expressing			
HLA-DR	24	—	18	—
CD38	32	—	81	—
CD57	41	—	42	—

can be one of two types. Ninety to 95% of T cells in normal adult peripheral blood express the alpha/beta heterodimer, and the rest express the gamma/delta heterodimer. In normal healthy adults, most gamma/delta-expressing T cells ($CD3^+$) do not express CD4 or CD8. This population is thus sometimes referred to as the $CD4^-$ $CD8^-$ T cells. In HIV infection, the gamma/delta T cells, including those that are $CD4^-$ $CD8^-$, are elevated.[28] In routine immunophenotyping, these cells may cause the CD3 percentage to be significantly higher than the sum of the CD4 + CD8 percentages.

NK Lymphocytes

Natural killer (NK) cells have been shown to lyse HIV-infected target cells in vitro. In addition, they are the effector cells for antibody-dependent cellular cytotoxicity and play a role in the first-line defense against a variety of pathogens. The number of NK cells measured by CD16 (Leu11) monoclonal antibody does not decrease during HIV disease despite a dramatic decrease in NK function during the later stages, that is, AIDS. It is generally believed that this decrease in function may reflect a failure of CD4 cell IL-2 production in vitro, because NK functional activity is restored in vitro by the addition of IL-2. With respect to cell-surface phenotype, recent reports have suggested that NK cells in HIV-infected people gradually lose CD16 and CD56 coexpression (29–31). This work is being extended now in several laboratories, and dual-color or three-color enumeration of NK cell phenotype is likely to prove prognostically useful as an adjunct to T-cell assessments currently in place.

B Lymphocytes

Average B-cell percentages and absolute numbers are decreased in the circulation of HIV-infected people compared to normal healthy controls, but these values are seldom outside the normal range. In AIDS, there are more immature B cells, and a few express common acute lymphocytic leukemia antigen (CALLA) CD10.[32] There are also activated B cells that spontaneously secrete immunoglobulin. Although B-cell enumeration is important to complete the immunophenotyping panel, prognostic significance has not been associated with specific B-cell alterations at various stages of HIV disease.

Direct Measurements of Viral Load

A direct measure of viral load is required for optimal monitoring of HIV-infected individuals. Such monitoring could then delineate the natural history of the infection as well as assess the effectiveness of new antiretroviral therapies.

Viral load has three major components: cell-free virus; infected cells, containing both actively replicating virus and viral components; and cells containing proviral DNA. The existence of all these compartments possibly distributed throughout the body makes this measurement quite difficult. One practical approach is to assume that the viral load in the peripheral blood will reflect the viral load of the entire body.

Initial experiments of Harper et al.[33] suggested that very few peripheral blood cells were infected by HIV. Using in situ hybridization techniques, they found viral RNA in 86% (6 of 7) of lymph nodes examined and in only 50% (7 of 14) of peripheral blood samples examined. Labeled cells were seen at a very low frequency (<0.01% of total mononuclear cells). Viral RNA was estimated at between 20 and 300 copies per cell.

Consensus protocols for viral culture have been adopted by many laboratories, for example, those involved in the AIDS Clinical Trials Group, and allow measurement not only of cells actively replicating HIV but also of cells induced to produce virus from proviral DNA. Recent attempts to quantify free virus, as well as actively infected cells[34,35] have been successful. Interestingly, the number of infectious viral particles or infected peripheral blood cells found is substantially higher (1 of 4,000) than those estimated by Harper et al.[33] If one takes the mean number of infected cells (2,200/10^6 cells for AIDS patients; range, 50–100,000) and divides it by the fraction of CD4-bearing cells, assumed to be 10% of the lymphocytes, one can infer that 1 in 40 (2.5%) of the CD4-bearing lymphocytes could be infected. If one assumes that $CD4^+$ cells represent only 1% of the lymphocytes in these AIDS patients, 25% of the $CD4^+$ lymphocytes could be infected. Should the percentage of $CD4^+$ fall by another factor of 4, virtually all $CD4^+$ lymphocytes could be infected.

The rapid rate of analysis of cells by flow cytometry (approaching 6,000 cells) allows relatively rare events, such as the circulating HIV-infected cell, to be sought using this technology. As an example, it would take 16.7 minutes to evaluate 1,000,000 cells at 1,000 cells per second. Thus it is potentially feasible to quantify HIV-infected cells present at 0.01% of the peripheral blood mononuclear cells, as suggested by Harper et al.[33] Flow cytometry is the method of choice, because of the rapid rate (approaching 6,000 cell/sec if necessary) at which cells can be analyzed and because correlated multiparametric analysis of large databases is feasible with this technology.

Cell Sorting

Schnittman and colleagues[36] used cell sorting to obtain specific subsets of circulating lymphocytes from infected individuals based on their cell-surface phenotype. They performed PCR assays on various dilutions of the sorted CD4-bearing cells. All the PCR positivity was found in CD4-bearing cells, and indications were that approximately 1% of the CD4-

bearing cells contained HIV proviral DNA. Psallidopoulos et al.[37] performed similar experiments using samples from seropositive asymptomatic individuals. Again, the major population of infected cells was the CD4$^+$ lymphocyte, found in all 10 samples. Estimates indicated that between 1 in 100 and 1 in 40,000 CD4$^+$ cells were infected, depending on the individual. Again, a small signal was occasionally obtained from the CD4$^-$ lymphocytes. These investigators suggested a viral load in four of their asymptomatic individuals (1/100 CD4$^+$ cells) very similar to the burden found in individuals with AIDS.

These investigators and others[36,38] thus suggested that the number of circulating HIV-infected cells is considerably higher than previously reported. Also, Schnittman et al. contended that the CD4-bearing lymphocyte is the principal reservoir of HIV infection. Further, because of the distribution of anti-CD4 antibody binding per lymphocyte, it appears that the vast majority of infected cells have not downregulated CD4, although such downregulation has been observed after experimental infections. A similar conclusion was drawn by Walker et al.,[39] who found HIV associated with CD4$^+$ cells selected from peripheral blood mononuclear cells by panning.

More recently Schnittman and colleagues have evaluated the infection of specific subsets of CD4-bearing lymphocytes.[40] They found that the infection occurs preferentially, although not exclusively, in the CD4$^+$CD45RO$^+$ subset. This phenotype marks the "memory" cells. This observation may help to explain two previously puzzling observations. First, in young children with HIV disease, *Pneumocystis carinii* pneumonia may occur when CD4 counts are well over 1,000/mm^3. It will be interesting to establish what fraction of these remaining cells are CD45RO$^+$, because young children may well have an oversupply of "virgin" CD4$^+$CD45RA$^+$ cells. The second dilemma arises in trying to reconcile the downregulation of CD4 seen in culture with the data of Schnittman et al. suggesting that such downregulation does not occur in vivo. Here again, the bulk of the remaining CD4$^+$ cells may be CD45RA$^+$, the phenotype that is less likely to be infected with HIV and thus less likely to show downregulation.

Cell-Associated p24 Antigen

Lymphocyte p24-FCA is a new flow-cytometric test[41] that quantifies circulating lymphocytes which contain actively replicating HIV (Figure 9.5). The test relies for its specificity on a MAb that binds to the HIV core antigen p24 (or p25). The assumption is made that the presence of cytoplasmic HIV p24 antigen indicates active viral protein synthesis. Binding to the MAb is revealed by indirect immunofluorescence after fixation of the cells to allow entrance of the MAb. The number of lymphocytes containing actively replicating HIV is quantified by flow

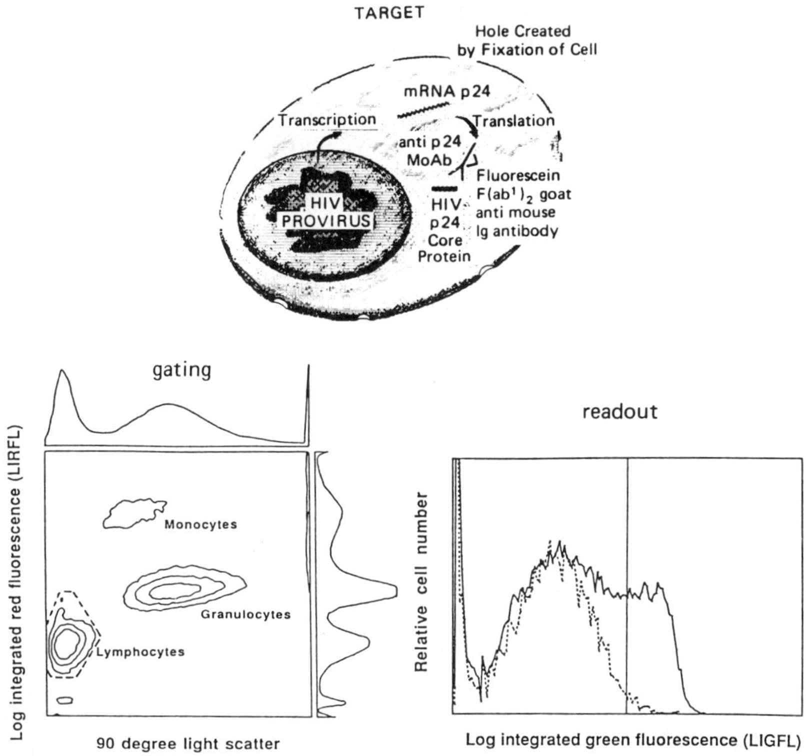

FIGURE 9.5. Lymphocyte p24-FCA. Target for p24 flow-cytometric analysis is a fixed, permeabilized, HIV-infected, peripheral blood lymphocyte. Binding of HIV p24- (p25-) specific murine monoclonal antibody (MAb) is revealed by indirect immunofluorescence as indicated in top panel and quantified by flow cytometry using lymphocyte analysis region to identify cells with low-angle light scatter and low binding of CD14-specific MAb as lymphocytes (gating panel, life). Histograms show green fluorescence of positive (16.4%) (——) and negative (0.1%) (----) population of lymphocytes in readout panel (right).

cytometry and expressed as the number of lymphocytes that are p24-antigen positive (p24$^+$). In model systems, this test detects 1 HIV-infected lymphoblastoid cells among 10^4 uninfected cells.[42]

Direct comparisons of lymphocyte p24-FCA data from the same peripheral blood samples used for viral culture were made.[41] A strong inverse relationship between positive lymphocyte p24-FCA results and the number of days required to obtain a positive viral culture was observed.

Comparison of asymptomatic, HIV-seropositive, serum p24 antigen-negative individuals to patients with AIDS either untreated or receiving zidovudine therapy showed that the range of values for asymptomatic individuals was remarkably similar to that seen in untreated individuals with AIDS. Individuals receiving zidovudine therapy showed a much lower range of values than did the other two study groups.[41] The same similar pencentage of infected lymphocytes in asymptomatic individuals and individuals with AIDS was observed by Psallidopoulos et al.[37]

Again, the number of circulating virus-infected lymphocytes as revealed by lymphocyte p24-FCA was high, in some cases approaching 25% of all circulating lymphocytes. Calculation of the ratio of $p24^+$ lymphocytes to $CD4^+$ lymphocytes revealed some interesting facts. First, the ratio was quite low (<0.5) in 53 of 55 asymptomatic individuals, consistent with the idea that infection is confined to only a limited number of the CD4-bearing lymphocytes. Second, 2 of 55 who had ratios between 0.5 and 1.0 differed from the rest of the study group in that they progressed to AIDS within 2 weeks of testing.

Interestingly, a direct comparison of the lymphocyte p24-FCA data from the same sample used for viral culture indicated a strong inverse relationship between positive lymphocyte p24-FCA results and the number of days required to obtain a positive viral culture.

Recent longitudinal studies show that HIV replication appears to progress in recurring episodes of intense viral replication involving large numbers of cells actively replicating the virus interspersed with periods of relative quiescence, where the number of cells actively replicating HIV falls below the level of detection possible with lymphocyte p24-FCA. Late in the infection it appears that some $CD4^-$ lymphocytes may become infected in certain individuals. The identity of these cells remains to be established.

Other investigators have also employed flow cytometry to quantify HIV-infected peripheral blood cells. McSharry and his colleagues[43] performed a cross-sectional study using peripheral blood mononuclear cells from individuals with HIV disease. Their approach differed slightly from that described previously in that they measured binding of monoclonal antibodies directed against HIV as a function of the DNA content of the peripheral blood mononuclear cells. They also found quite high numbers (as high as 24%) of cells that were positive for HIV-nef or HIV-p24. A significant correlation was demonstrated ($p = 0.0001$) between the CDC status of the patients and the percentage of p24 antigen-positive mononuclear cells. No correlation was observed with serum p24 antigen.

Two different laboratories have thus found flow cytometry to provide a direct measure of the cell-associated component of viral load in peripheral blood.

Potential Usefulness of Direct Measures of Viral Load

Monitoring individuals with HIV disease should be aided by use of lymphocyte p24-FCA or other direct measures of cells actively replicating HIV. The current first line of defense, zidovudine, has some associated toxicity to bone marrow, and these side effects continue to accrue as long as zidovudine is given. Because zidovudine inhibits HIV reverse transcriptase and is thus only active against the initial stages of HIV infection of cells, it would seem prudent to treat with the drug only when the viral infection is active. Thus use of this test may define appropriate treatment periods and, by allowing certain periods of recovery from unwanted side effects when the viral infection is relatively quiescent, may extend the period of time during which a given individual can be treated with zidovudine.

Another potential use of this technology is to assay for active viral replication in individuals for whom the standard serotests are not meaningful, for example, infants born to HIV-seropositive mothers who carry maternal antibody and individuals who may eventually receive an HIV vaccine. Preliminary data suggest that this technique may be able to detect infection in infants born to seropositive mothers,[44] but longitudinal follow-up is needed for confirmation.

Conclusions

Flow cytometric enumeration of lymphocyte subsets is an extremely valuable technology to aid in understanding the biology of HIV disease and in assessing the immune system of individual people during disease progression. With respect to the biology of HIV disease, three- and four-color immunofluorescence promises to add further to our knowledge. Cell-sorting experiments to test the function of phenotypic subsets is under way. With respect to patient care, additional studies and analysis of existing data, especially in conjunction with soluble markers of immune activation including neopterin, beta$_2$-microglobulin, and p24, are being conducted to improve the utility of CD4 T-lymphocyte measurements for staging HIV disease, selecting participants for trials, and monitoring therapy. Newer flow cytometry systems promise to simplify quality control and guarantee increased accuracy and reproducibility of results. Finally, the widespread need for more economical means of obtaining T-lymphocyte subset values, including CD4 levels, should drive furter development and maturation of clinical flow-cytometric immunophenotyping.

Acknowledgments. The gracious assistance of Ms. Lisa Doster and Ms. Lisa Wilhelm in the preparation of this manuscript and Ms. Elizabeth Steck in the preparation of the figures is gratefully acknowledged. One of us (BMOW) was partially supported by a contract N01-HB-67023, Project 221924 from the National Heart, Lung, and Blood Institute; the other (ALL) was supported in part by U01-AI25915 from the National Institute for Allergy and Infectious Disease.

References

1. Loken MR, Stall AM. Flow cytometry as an analytical and preparative tool in immunology. J Immunol Methods 1982;50:85–112.
2. Parks DR, Herzenberg LA. Fluorescence-activated cell sorting: theory, experimental optimization, and applications in lymphoid cell biology. Methods Enzymol 1984;108:197–241.
3. Shapiro HM. Practical Flow Cytometry. New York: Alan R. Liss, 1988.
4. Levi FA, Cannon C, Tonitoe Y, Reinberg A, and Mathe G. Seasonal modulation of the circadian time structure of circulating T and natural killer lymphocyte subsets for healthy subjects. J Clin Invest 1988;81:407–413.
5. Paxton H, Kidd P, Landay A, Giorgi J, Flomenberg N, Walker E. Results of the flow cytometry ACTG quality control program: analysis and findings. Clin Immunol Immunopathol 1989;52:68–85.
6. Thornthwaite JT, Rosenthal PK, Vazquez DA, Seckinger D. The effects of anticoagulant and temperature on the measurement of helper and suppressor cells. Diagn Immunol 1984;2:167–174.
7. Weiblen BJ, Debell K, Valeri CR. "Acquired immunodeficiency" of blood stored overnight. N Engl J Med 1983;309:793.
8. Ashmore LM, Shopp GM, Edwards BS. Lymphocyte subset analysis by flow cytometry comparison of three different staining techniques and effects of blood storage. J Immunol Methods 1989;118:209–215.
9. Giorgi JV. Lymphocyte subset measurements: significance in clinical medicine. In Fahey JL, Friedman H, Rose NR, eds. Manual of Clinical Laboratory Immunology. Washington DC: American Society for Microbiology, 1986:236–246.
10. Workshop antigen designation. J Immunol 1989;143:758–759.
11. Knapp W, Rieber P, Dorken B, Schmidt RE, Stein H, Borne AEGV. Towards a better definition of human leukocyte surface molecules. Immunol Today 1989;10:253–258.
12. Landay A, Muirhead K. Procedural guidelines for performing immunophenotyping by flow cytometry. Clin Immunol Immunopath 1989;52:48–60.
13. Loken MR, Bronman JM, Bach BA, Ault KA. Quality control in flow cytometry. I. establishing optimal gates for immunophenotyping. Cytometry 1990;11:453–459.
14. Liu CM, Muirhead KA, George SP, Landay AL. Flow cyteometric monitoring of human immunodeficiency virus infected patients: simultaneous enumeration of five lymphocyte subsets. Am J Clin Pathol 1989;92:721–728.
15. National Committee for Clinical Laboratory Standards. Clinical applications of flow cytometry quality assurance and immunophenotyping of peripheral blood lymphocytes. NCCLS Publ. H42-P. Villanove, Pennslyluania: NCCLS, 1989.
16. Zolla-Pazner S, DesJarlais DC, Friedlan SR, Spira TJ, Marmor M, Holzman R. Mildvan D, Yancovitz S, Mathur-Wagh U, Garber J, El-Sadr W, Cohen H, Smith D, Kalyanaraman VS, Kaplan JE, Fishbein DB. Non-random development of immunologic abnormalities after infection with human immunodeficiency virus: implications for immunologic classification of the disease. Proc Natl Acad Sci USA 1987;84:5405–5408.

17. Kaslow RA, Ostrow DG, Detels R, Phair JP, Polk BF, Rinaldo CR. The multicenter AIDS cohort study: rationale, organization, and selected characteristics of the participants. Am J Epidemiol 1987;126:310–318.
18. Giorgi JV, Nishanian PG, Schmid I, Hultin LE, Cheng H, Detels R. Selective alterations in immunoregulatory lymphocyte subsets in early HIV (human T-lymphotropic virus type II/lymphadenopathy-associated virus) infection. J Clin Immunol 1987;7:140–150.
19. Giorgi JV, Fahey JL, Smith DC, Hultin LE, Cheng H-L, Mitsuyasu RT, Detels R. Early effects of HIV on CD4 lymphocytes in vivo. J Immunol 1987;138:3725–3730.
20. Giorgi JV, Detels R. T-cell subset alterations in HIV-infected homosexual men: NIAID multicenter AIDS cohort study. Clin Immunol Immunopathol 1989;52:10–18.
21. Lang W, Perkins H, Anderson R, Royce R, Jewell N, Winkelstein W. Patterns of T-lymphocyte changes with human immunodeficiency virus infection: from seroconversion to development of AIDS. J Acquir Immune Defic Syndr 1989;2:63–69.
22. Taylor JMG, Fahey JL, Detels R, Giorgi JV. CD4 percentage, CD4 number and CD4:CD8 ratio in HIV infection: which to choose and how to use. J Acquir Immune Defic Syndr 1989;2:114–124.
23. Fletcher MA, Azen SP, Adelsberg B, Gjerset G, Hassett J, Kaplan J, Niland JC, Odom-Maryon T, Parker JW, Stites DP, Mosley JW, and Transfusion Safety Group. Immunophenotyping in a multicenter study: the transfusion safety study experience. Clin Immunol Immunopathol, 1989;52:38–47.
24. Nicholson JKA, McDougal JS, Spira TJ, Croas GD, Jones BM, Reinherz EL. Immunoregulatory subsets of the T helper and T suppressor cell populations in homosexual men with chronic unexplained lymphadenopathy. J Clin Invest 1984;73:191–201.
25. Nicholson JKA, McDougal JS, Jaffe HW, Spira TJ, Kennedy MS, Jones BM, Darrow WW, Morgan M, Hubbard M. Exposure to human T-lymphotropic virus type III/lymphadenopathy-associated virus and immunologic abnormalities in asymptomatic homosexual men. Ann Intern Med 1985;103:37–42.
26. Bach BA, Campbell D, Robertson MJ, Ullery S, Borowitz MJ. T-cell activation markers (HLA-DR, CD38, CD35, CD69) are expressed discordantly in HIV infected individuals. Blood 1989;74:339a.
27. Sites DP, Casavant CH, McHugh TM, Moss AR, Beal SL, Ziegler JL, Saunders AM, Warner NL. Flow cytometric analysis of lymphocyte phenotypes in AIDS using monoclonal antibodies and simultaneous dual immunofluorescence. Clin Immunol Immunopathol 1986;38:161–177.
28. Margolick JB, Carey V, Munoz A, Polk BF, Giorgi JV, Bauer KD, Kaslow R, Rinaldo C. Development of antibodies to HIV-1 is associated with an increase in circulating $CD3^+$ $CD4^-$ $CD8^-$ lymphocytes. Clin Immunol Immunopathol 1989;51:348–861.
29. Vuillier F, Bianco NE, Montagnier L, Dighiero G. Selective depletion of low density $CD8^+$, $CD16^+$ lymphocytes during HIV infection. AIDS Res Hum Retrovir 1988;4:121–129.
30. Ojo-Amaize E, Nishanian PG, Heitjan DF, Rezal A, Esmail I, Korns E, Detels R. Fahey J, Giorgi JV. Serum and effector-cell antibody-dependent cellular cytotoxicity (ADCC) activity remains high during human immunodeficiency virus (HIV) disease progression. J Clin Immunol 1989;9:454–461.

31. Robinson WE, Mitchell WM, Chambers WH, Schuftman SS, Montefiori DC, Oeltmann TW. Natural killer cell infection and inactivation in vitro by the human immunodeficiency virus. Hum Pathol 1988;19:535–540.
32. Martinez-Maza O, Crabb E, Mitsuyasu RT, Fahey JL, Giorgi JV. Infection with the human immunodeficiency virus (HIV) is associated with an *in vivo* increase in B lymphocyte activation and immaturity. Immunol 1987;138: 3720–3724.
33. Harper ME, Marselle LM, Gallo RC, Wong-Stall F. Detection of T lymphocytes expressing human T-lymphotropic virus type III in lymph node and peripheral blood from infected individuals by in situ hybridization. Proc Natl Acad Sci USA 1986;83:772–776.
34. Ho DD, Moughi T, and Alam M. Quantitation of HIV-1 in the blood of infected persons. N Engl J Med 1989;321:1621–1625.
35. Coombs RW, Collier AC, Allain JP, Nikora B, Leuther M, Gjerset GF, Corey L. Plasma viremia in human immunodeficiency virus infection. N Engl J Med 1989;321:1626–1631.
36. Schnittman, SM, Psallidopoulos MC, Lane C, Thompson L, Baseler M, Massari F, Fox CH, Salzman P, Fauci AS. The reservoir for HIV-1 in human peripheral blood is a T cell that maintains expression of CD4. Science 1989;245:305–308.
37. Psallidopoulos, MC, Schnittman SM, Thompson III LM, Baseler M, Fauci AS, Lane HC, Salzman NP. Integrated proviral human immunodeficiency virus type 1 is present in $CD4^+$ peripheral blood lymphocytes in healthy seropositive individuals. J of Virology 1989;63:4626–4631.
38. Ulrich, PP, Busch MP, El-Beik T, et al. Assessment of human immunodeficiency virus expression in cocultures of PBMCs from healthy seropositive individuals. J Med Virol 1988;75:1–10.
39. Walker, CM, Moody DJ, Stites DP, Levy JA. $CD8^+$ T lymphocyte control of HIV replication in cultured $CD4^+$ cell varies among infected individuals. Cell Immunol 1989;119:470–475.
40. Schnittman, SM, Clifford Lane, H, Greenhouse J, Justement JS, Baseler M, Fauci AS. Preferential infection of $CD4^+$ memory T cells by human immunodeficiency virus type 1: Evidence for a role in the selective T-cell functional defects observed in infected individuals. Proc Natl Acad Sci USA 1990;87: 6058–6062.
41. Ohlsson-Wilhelm, BM, Cory JM, Kessler HA, Eyster ME, Rapp F, Landay A. Circulating HIV p24 antigen-positive lymphocytes: a flow cytometric measure of HIV infection. J Infect Dis 1990;162:1018–1024.
42. Cory, JM, Ohlsson-Wilhelm BM, Brock EJ, Shaeffer NA, Steck ME, Eyster ME. Rapp F. Detection of human immunodeficiency virus infected lymphoid cells of low frequency by flow cytometry. J Immunol Methods 1987;105: 71–78.
43. McSharry JJ, Constantino R, Robblano E, Echols R, Stevens R, Lehman JM. Detection and quantification of HIV-infected peripheral blood mononuclear cells by flow cytometry. J Clin Micro 1990;28(4):724–733.
44. Rich, KC, Cory JM, Landay AL, Ohlsson-Wilhelm BM. Lymphocyte associated p24 antigen: a new technique for diagnosis of HIV infection in pediatric patients. 6th Int Conf AIDS, San Francisco CA 1990;3:320.

10
Prognostic Indicators for Progression of HIV Disease

C. Robert Horsburgh

Infection with the human immunodeficiency virus (HIV) produces a prolonged, gradually progressive illness that eventually leads to opportunistic infections, malignancy, and death. The illness may last 10 years or longer and is usually asymptomatic for the first several years. Over time, the immune system gradually weakens, and clinical signs and symptoms become apparent. However, the course of the illness is quite variable from individual to individual, both in its duration and in its clinical and laboratory manifestations.

It would be useful to have prognostic indicators of the progression of HIV disease, both to aid clinicians and patients in coping with the illness and to allow evaluation of the effect of therapeutic interventions. A number of markers of disease stage have been identified: these include clinical syndromes, immunologic laboratory parameters, and virologic laboratory parameters. Most of these have been evaluted prospectively and found to correlate with the risk of progression to AIDS, as defined in the Centers for Disease Control (CDC) case definition, while a few have been shown to predict survival as well.

Use of AIDS as an endpoint in validating prognostic indicators for HIV disease introduces some difficulties, because the occurrence of an opportunistic infection or malignancy requires both exposure and susceptibility. Thus two individuals who are at the same stage of disease may acquire AIDS at different times if one is exposed to an opportunistic pathogen and the other is not. Moreover, the AIDS case definition is heterogeneous; some AIDS-defining conditions occur at a time when immunologic impairment is minimal while others only occur when impairment is severe. Persons who present with Kaposi's sarcoma have a significantly longer survival than those who present with *Pneumocystis carinii* pneumonia (PCP), confirming that these two AIDS-indicating diagnoses are not equivalent. However, because studies of prognostic indicators with survival as the endpoint must wait additional years before analysis, most studies of prognostic markers of HIV disease have used AIDS as the outcome variable.

The prolonged course of HIV disease has also made it difficult to identify early markers for progression. Even if AIDS rather than death is used as the endpoint, little information is available from persons who were infected with HIV during the early years of the HIV epidemic, and few persons who were in the early stages of HIV infection in the mid-1980s have progressed to AIDS; thus, most of the markers that have been defined are those that indicate moderate to severe disease. It is hoped that earlier prognostic indicators will be defined in the coming years.

Last, although a large number of markers for disease progression have been identified, the prognostic value of multiple markers cannot be assumed to be additive. Thus, the clinician will need to determine which markers might be of value for an individual patient. A few studies have examined the interactions between various markers, but no study has examined the entire range of proposed indicators. The final section of this chapter examines some of these interactions and makes some general recommendations.

Clinical Markers

A number of clinical conditions have been shown to be associated with HIV infection. Among the first manifestations to appear after HIV infection are the acute retroviral syndrome, generalized lymphadenopathy, and a distinctive dermatitis resembling seborrheic dermatitis. While early reports suggested that generalized lymphadenopathy was a significant marker of disease progression, more recent studies have shown that this syndrome does not predict subsequent progression to AIDS.[1–3] Moreover, the resolution of such lymphadenopathy, which had been considered a grave sign, has not been confirmed as a prognostic indicator. Neither the presence or absence of an acute retroviral syndrome, nor of dermatitis, has been shown to relate to the eventual course of disease. However, as noted, this may result from the difficulty in recognizing the value of such early signs at our present place in the epidemic. It is hoped that studies confirming or refuting the value of such signs in prognosis of HIV infection will be forthcoming.

Several later clinical conditions have been recognized to be indicators of a more rapid progression to AIDS. The first of these to be recognized was the presence of oral mucocutaneous candidiasis (thrush). Several studies have confirmed that HIV-infected persons with thrush have a significantly increased risk of developing AIDS.[4,5] Although less common, an episode of herpes zoster also appears to herald a more rapid occurrence of AIDS.[6] Third, the presence of oral hairy leukoplakia (OHL), an infection of the tongue or oral cavity with Epstein–Barr virus, also is associated with subsequent development of AIDS.[7] Of these three conditions, thrush is the most useful indicator, and has been evaluated in several of the combined systems (see *Staging Systems*). OHL appears to be of limited value as a marker because it is reported infrequently in many populations. This may be because it is often asymptomatic and therefore may not be clinically recognized.

Two other conditions that represent significant illness in HIV-infected individuals are bacterial pneumonia and pulmonary tuberculosis. Several authors have suggested that the occurrence of one of these illnesses may predict subsequent AIDS, but prospective studies to confirm these suspicions have not been reported.

Immunologic Markers

Early in the HIV epidemic it was recognized that HIV infection is characterized by progressive, irreversible decline of the helper T-lymphocyte population. These cells are essential for proper immunologic response to many pathogens, and their destruction is thought to be the explanation for the increased susceptibility of HIV-infected persons to fungal, viral, and parasitic pathogens. The cells are distinguished by the presence on their surface of an antigenic protein called CD4 (previously known as T4 or Leu3). Such cells are identified by staining with antibodies to CD4; this is usually performed with a cytofluorometer (see Chapter 9, this volume). The result is expressed as the percent of peripheral blood mononuclear cells that are CD4 positive. In the HIV-uninfected person, 20–40% of cells are CD4 positive.

The percent of CD4-positive cells is commonly multiplied by the absolute lymphocyte count to produce a "helper T-cell count." This value is usualy 500–1,500 cells/cubic millimeter in the absence of HIV infection. The daily variability and interlaboratory variability of this parameter is considerable because of fluctuations in white blood cell count and differential.[8] For this reason, some authors have advocated relying on helper cell percentage rather than absolute number.[8–10] However, while the helper cell percentage is somewhat more accurate and reproducible, the two indices are clinically interchangable, and the absolute $CD4^+$ cell count has more widespread usage.

The $CD4^+$ cell count has been shown in a number of studies to be the strongest prognostic indicator for both AIDS and survival. Because of this, it is widely obtained and used in the clinical setting. It appears that the $CD4^+$ count declines gradually at a rate of about 80 cells per year from the time of HIV infection to a level of 400–500/mm^3.[11] At that point the decline may become more precipitous, although this is not always the case. Because zidovudine has been shown to decrease the occurrence of AIDS in persons with 500 or fewer $CD4^+$ cells,[12,13] it is now recommended that zidovudine therapy be initiated when the $CD4^+$ count falls below 500/mm^3. Although some persons will show a transient rise in $CD4^+$ counts after beginning zidovudine, $CD4^+$ counts will continue to fall. Counts should be monitored every 6 months; when they reach $200/mm^3$, prophylactic therapy for PCP should be initiated.[14]

The suppressor T-lymphocyte population ($CD8^+$) is also affected by HIV infection. In acute HIV infection, $CD8^+$ cells rise and then return to normal over a period of months. Then, as HIV infection persists, $CD8^+$ cell numbers decline, although not as rapidly as $CD4^+$ cells. This decline is often expressed as a helper/suppressor ratio ($CD4^+$:$CD8^+$). While this ratio is also a prognostic indicator for HIV disease, it is less specific than the $CD4^+$ cell count and has been largely replaced by it.[9] Evaluation of $CD8^+$ cell counts has not been shown to provide useful prognostic information.

Because enumeration of $CD4^+$ cells requires expensive laboratory equipment and specially trained technicians, efforts have been made to find serum markers of immunologic status that could substitute for the $CD4^+$ count. The most successful of these is the assay of beta$_2$-microglobulin (B_2M). B_2M is a lymphocyte surface protein that is released into the serum by destruction of cells. Thus, as $CD4^+$ cell counts fall, B_2M levels rise. Normal B_2M values are less than 2 mg/l, while persons with symptomatic HIV infection may have 4–5 mg/l. However, B_2M levels reflect turnover of all lymphocytes and are thus inherently less specific than $CD4^+$ cell counts. Moreover, B_2M levels rise with age in the normal population and may be elevated by intravenous drug use, limiting their usefulness in some HIV-infected populations.

Nonetheless, as a predictor of prognosis of HIV disease, B_2M is nearly as accurate as the $CD4^+$ count.[3,14] The combination of the two tests improves the prognostic accuracy of either test alone. At the present time, however, no B_2M values have been established to indicate therapeutic thresholds such as exist for $CD4^+$ cell counts.

Serum neopterin levels have also been evaluated as a prognostic indicator of HIV disease.[15] Neopterin, a metabolite of dihydroneopterin triphosphate, is produced from guanosine triphosphate (GTP) when cells of the immune system are activated. The average serum neopterin level in the HIV-uninfected individual is 5 nmol/l, but in HIV-infected persons the average is nearly 14 nmol/l. Neopterin levels are not as useful in prognosis as $CD4^+$ counts, but, as with B_2M, the combination of $CD4^+$ and neopterin is more accurate than either alone.[15]

Several other soluble proteins that are products of immune activation have also been shown to have abnormal values in advanced HIV infection, but these either have not been confirmed as prognostic indicators or have not yet been prospectively studied. They include serum interferon alpha, soluble CD4, soluble CD8, and soluble interleukin-2 receptor.

Although total immunoglobulin levels, and particularly IgA levels, rise precipitously after HIV infection, their prognostic usefulness is unclear. A few studies have suggested that persons with higher IgA levels had a more rapid progression to AIDS,[15,16] but measurement of this parameter has not added significantly to other indicators of disease progression.

HIV infection results in the production of antibodies to a number of HIV proteins, and several of these antibodies have been investigated as possible prognostic indicators. These include antibody to the p24 core protein, antibody to reverse transcriptase, antibodies to the envelope protein gp120, and antibodies to specific envelope regions such as the principal neutralizing domain or a portion of the gp41 moiety. The most widely investigated has been antibody to p24, which appears to decline before the development of AIDS.[16–18] This has been shown in some studies to have prognostic value in addition to the CD4$^+$ count. Reports of the prognostic value of antibodies to the envelope protein and to specific envelope regions remain to be confirmed.

In general, while abnormalities of in vitro mitrogen proliferation such as to phytohemagglutinin, concanavalin A, or pokeweed mitogen are commonly reported to be abnormal in AIDS patients, their usefulness as prognostic indicators has been limited. This is the result of the concordance in most cases of these defects with severely depressed CD4$^+$ cell counts. Thus, in vitro mitogen stimulation assays do not usually give additional prognostic information.

On the other hand, HIV-infected persons may have defects in the ability of their lymphocytes to respond to antigen in vitro before significant decreases in CD4$^+$ cells occur. This has led several groups of investigators to evaluate such tests as prognostic indicators for HIV disease.[19–22] Such tests include antigen-stimulated lymphocyte proliferation, antigen-stimulated lymphokine production, and lymphocyte proliferation to anti-CD3. Decreased responsiveness to these assays has correlated with increased risk of progression to AIDS. However, it is not yet known whether such in vitro tests will add significantly to the predictive value of CD4$^+$ cell counts. Moreover, these tests are expensive, cumbersome, and time consuming to perform. Thus their role in clinical evaluation of HIV disease will probably remain limited.

Skin testing for determination of anergy has been proposed as an in vivo assessment of the ability of the immune system to respond to antigen stimulation and has the advantage of being inexpensive and simple to perform.[23] However, the test requires that patients return in 48 hours for reading; the difficulty of accomplishing this has led most investigators to omit this test.

Virologic Markers

Cross-sectional studies have suggested that the viral burden of the HIV-infected host increases over time. Thus, laboratory quantitation of the amount of HIV present might be expected to be a useful prognostic indicator. Several methods are available for virus detection, including antigen detection, virus culture, and polymerase chain reaction (PCR). The most extensively evaluated has been the p24 antigen assay.

Antigen to the core protein p24 can be detected and quantified using commercially available kits. Antigen can be detected before antibody appears in some patients and then may reappear in late-stage disease; in rare patients it persists throughout infection. The presence of antigen after detection of antibody correlates with more rapid progression to AIDS.[3,15,18] However, no relationship has been demonstrated between p24 antigen titer and disease progression. In one study where p24 antigen was evaluated along with $CD4^+$ counts and other indicators, antigen detection added little to prognostic ability,[15] while in another there was additional predictive value.[3] The lack of utility of antigen detection appears to be related to the relative insensitivity of the test; high levels of antigen in serum are needed for a positive test result. Such high levels most commonly occur at late stages of disease; at this time $CD4^+$ counts and other prognostic indicators are also markedly abnormal. More sensitive HIV antigen assays may increase the prognostic usefulness of antigen detection.

The amount of virus present in infected individuals can also be assessed by quantitative culture. Quantitative culture of HIV in plasma has recently been reported to correlate with stage of HIV disease.[24] However, this technique has not been evaluated to determine whether specific levels of plasma viremia have prognostic value. Moreover, the technique is expensive and time consuming. Because more than 90% of HIV-infected persons will have a positive peripheral blood virus culture, nonquantitative culture has little prognostic value.

Evaluation and quantitation of HIV DNA using PCR technology has recently been developed and shows promise in prognosis of HIV disease. A recent report has demonstrated that the number of copies of HIV DNA in peripheral blood of HIV-infected persons increases with advancing disease.[25] Whether such quantitation will be useful in prognosis of HIV disease remains to be determined.

Staging HIV Disease

As we have seen, many clinical, immunologic, and virologic markers have prognostic value in HIV disease. The single most predictive marker is the $CD4^+$ cell count; the value of other markers must be evaluated in terms of what additional prognostic value they add to $CD4^+$ counts. Prospective studies of various laboratory markers have shown that B_2M, serum neopterin, and p24 antigen assay add to the predictive value of $CD4^+$ counts, but the information gained for a particular patient is small. In the clinic at Grady Memorial Hospital in Atlanta, $CD4^+$ cell counts are the only laboratory marker routinely obtained.

TABLE 10.1. Parameters that may predict progression of HIV disease.

Clinical	Immunologic	Virologic
Thrush	$CD4^+$ cell counts or percentage	p24 antigen
Oral hairy leukoplakia	$Beta_2$-microglobulin	Quantitative plasma culture
Herpes zoster	Neopterin	Quantitative PCR
Bacterial pneumonia	Total IgA	
Pulmonary tuberculosis	p24 antibody	
Weight loss	Skin testing	

Of the clinical conditions, thrush is the most useful indicator that a patient needs more careful observation, even when $CD4^+$ counts are not severely depressed. I also note episodes of herpes zoster, oral hairy leukoplakia (OHL), bacterial pneumonia, and pulmonary tuberculosis as clinical indications of disease progression (Table 10.1).

Several groups have recognized the need to combine the most promising clinical and laboratory markers into a staging system for HIV disease. An early staging system, the Walter Reed Classification System,[23] has had limited acceptance by many clinicians because it requires skin testing, which is not commonly performed. The World Health Organization has recently proposed a staging system that has both a clinical and a laboratory component (Table 10.2).[26] In this system, Stage 1 includes persons without symptoms or with only persistent generalized lymphadenopathy. Stage 2 includes greater than 10% weight loss, minor mucocutaneous manifestations, herpes zoster, or recurrent upper respiratory tract infections. Stage 3 includes greater than 10% weight loss, unexplained chronic diarrhea of more than 1 month duration, thrush, OHL, pulmonary tuberculosis, or severe bacterial infections. Stage 4 is AIDS as defined by CDC or being bedridden more than 50% of the day. Prospective evaluation of this system is presently in progress.

Several other systems have been proposed, but none is in widespread use. The major difficulty is that systems which require extensive laboratory evaluation soon become too complex to be clinically useful. $CD4^+$ cell counts are widely available in the United States and Europe and are

TABLE 10.2. World Health Organization proposed staging system for HIV infection and disease.

Laboratory axis		Clinical axis			
Total lymphocyte count or	$CD4^+$ count	Asymptomatic	Early	Intermediate	Late
>2000/mm^3	>500/mm^3	1A	2A	3A	4A
1000–2000	200–500	1B	2B	3B	4B
<1000	<200	1C	2C	3C	4C

an important parameter in management of HIV disease in those areas. However, it is important to emphasize that even the $CD4^+$ count, by far the strongest predictor of the course of disease, can only provide the clinician and patient with a rough estimate of the risk of disease progression.

References

1. El-Sadr W, Marmor M, Zolla-Parner S, et al. Four-year prospective study of homosexual men: correlation of immunologic abnormalities, clinical status, and serology to human immunodeficiency virus. J Infect Dis 1987;155:789–793.
2. Lang W, Anderson RE, Perkins H, Grant RM, Lyman D, et al. Clinical, immunologic, and serologic findings in men at risk for acquired immunodeficiency syndrome. JAMA 1987;257:326–330.
3. Moss AR, Bacchetti P, Osmond D, Krampf W, Chaisson RE, et al. Seropositivity for HIV and the development of AIDS or AIDS related condition: three-year follow up of the San Francisco General Hospital cohort. Br Med J 1988;296:745–750.
4. Klein RS, Harris CA, Small CB, et al. Oral candidiasis in high-risk patients as the initial manifestation of the acquired immunodeficiency syndrome. N Engl J Med 1984;311:354–358.
5. Phair J, Munoz A, Detels R, Kaslow R, Rinaldo C, et al. The risk of *Pneumocystis carinii* pneumonia among men infected with human immunodeficiency virus type 1. N Engl J Med 1990;322:161–165.
6. Melbye M, Grossman RJ, Goedert JJ, Eyster EE, Biggar RJ. Risk of AIDS after herpes zoster. Lancet 1987;i:728–731.
7. Greenspan D, Greenspan JS, Hearst NG, et al. Relation of oral hairy leukoplakia to infection with the human immunodeficiency virus and the risk of developing AIDS. J Infect Dis 1987;155:475–481.
8. Malone JL, Simms TE, Gray GC, Wagner KF, Burge JR, et al. Sources of variability in repeated T-helper lymphocyte counts from human immunodeficiency virus type 1-infected patients: total lymphocyte count fluctuations and diurnal cycle are important. J Acquir Immune Defic Syndr 1990;3: 144–151.
9. Taylor JMG, Fahey JL, Detels R, Giorgi JV. CD4 percentage, CD4 number, and CD4:CD8 ratio in HIV infection: which to choose and how to use. J Acquir Immune Defic Syndr 1990;2:114–124.
10. Koepke JA, Landay AL. Precision and accuracy of absolute lymphocyte counts. Clin Immunol Immunopathol 1989;52:19–27.
11. Lang W, Perkins H, Anderson RE, Royce R, Jewell N, et al. Patterns of T-lymphocyte changes with human immunodeficiency virus infection: from seroconversion to the development of AIDS. J Acquir Immune Defic Syndr 1990;2:63–69.
12. Volberding PA, Lagakos SW, Koch MA, Pettinelli C, Myers MW, et al. Zidovudine in asymptomatic human immunodeficiency virus infection. N Engl J Med 1990;322:941–949.
13. Fischl MA, Richman DD, Hansen N, Collier AC, Carey JT, et al. The safety and efficacy of zidovudine in the treatment of subjects with mildly symptomatic human immunodeficiency virus type 1 infection. Ann Intern Med 1990;112:727–737.

14. Anonymous. Guidelines for prophylaxis against *Pneumocystis carinii* pneumonia for persons infected with human immunodeficiency virus. MMWR 1989;38:S1–S9.
15. Fahey JL, Taylor JMG, Detels R, Hoffman B, Melmed R et al. The prognostic value of cellular and serologic markers in infection with human immunodeficiency virus type 1. N Engl J Med 1990;322:166–172.
16. McDougal JS, Kennedy MS, Nicholson JKA, Spira TJ, Jaffe HW, et al. Antibody response to human immunodeficiency virus in homosexual men. Relation of antibody specificity, titer, and isotype to clinical status, severity of immunodeficiency, and disease progression. J Clin Invest 1987;80:316–324.
17. Weber JN, Clapham PR, Weiss RA, Parker D, Roberts C, et al. Human immunodeficiency virus infection in two cohorts of homosexual men: neutralising sera and association of anti-gag antibody with prognosis. Lancet 1987;i:119–122.
18. Lange JMA, Paul DA, Huisman HG, de Wolf F, van den Berg H, et al. Persistent HIV antigaenemia and decline of HIV core antibodies associated with transition to AIDS. Br Med J 1986;293:1459–1462.
19. Murray HW, Hillman JK, Rubin BY, Kelly CD, Jacobs JL, et al. Patients at risk for AIDS-related opportunistic infections. N Engl J Med 1985;313: 1504–1510.
20. Ballet J-J, Couderc L-J, Rabian-Herzog C, Duval-Roy C, Janier M, et al. Impaired T-lymphocyte-dependent immune responses to microbial antigens in patients with HIV-1-associated persistent generalized lymphadenopathy. AIDS 1988;2:291–297.
21. Hoffman B, Bygbjerg I, Dickmeiss E, Faber V, Frederiksen B, et al. Prognostic value of immunologic abnormalities and HIV antigenemia in asymptomatic HIV-infected individuals: proposal of immunologic staging. Scand J Infect Dis 1989;21:633–643.
22. Schellekens PTA, Roos MTL, DeWolf F, Lanse JMA, Miedema F. Low T-cell responsiveness to activation via CD3/TCR is a prognostic marker for acquired immunodeficiency syndrome in human immunodeficiency virus-1-infected men. J Clin Immunol 1990;2:121–127.
23. Redfield RR, Wright DC, Tramont EC. The Walter Reed staging classification for HTLV-III/LAV infection. N Engl J Med 1986;314:131–132.
24. Ho DD, Mougdil T, Alam M. Quantitation of human immunodeficiency virus type 1 in the blood of infected persons. N Engl J Med 1989;321: 1621–1625.
25. Schnittman SM, Greenhouse JJ, Psallidopoulos MC, Baseler M, Salzman NP, et al. Increasing viral burden in $CD4^+$ T cells from patients with human immunodeficiency virus infection reflects rapidly progressive immunosuppression and clinical. Ann Intern Med 1990;113:438–443.
26. Anonymous. Acquired immunodeficiency syndrome. Interim proposal for a WHO staging system for HIV infecton and disease. Wkly Epidemiol Rec 1990;65:221–228.

11
Human Immunodeficiency Virus Infection in Children

Martha F. Rogers and Gerald Schochetman

Children represent an increasingly important part of the human immunodeficiency virus (HIV) epidemic. As of December 31, 1990, 2,786 children under the age of 13 years had been reported to the Centers for Disease Control (CDC), representing 1.7% of all reported AIDS cases. In the past year, cases due to perinatal (mother-to-child) transmission had the largest increase in number of reported AIDS cases compared with all other transmission groups.[1] Prepubertal children acquire HIV primarily through two routes: (i) perinatally through exposure to their infected mothers and (ii) parenterally through transfusions of blood or blood products. Transmission through sexual abuse or through percutaneous exposure to contaminated needles used for illicit drug injection is possible but such are rarely reported. Of the 2,786 children reported, 2,327 (84%) acquired HIV perinatally, 252 (9%) acquired HIV through transfusion of blood or blood products, 139 (5%) were children with coagulation disorders, and 68 (2%) were children with undetermined modes of transmission (usually undetermined because of inadequate information).

The laboratory and clinical diagnosis of HIV infection in children presents some unique problems. Because of the passive transfer of maternal antibody in utero, HIV infection in infants born to HIV-infected mothers cannot be confirmed with the anti-HIV antibody assays commonly used for diagnosis in adults. Certain clinical features such as disease manifestations, incubation, and latency period to development of AIDS are different in children than in adults. Understanding these differences is important for diagnosing HIV infection in children. This chapter reviews the modes of transmission and clinical features of HIV infection and discusses laboratory diagnosis in the pediatric propulation.

Modes of Transmission in Children

Perinatal/Vertical Transmission

Because donor deferral and screening of the blood supply have virtually eliminated transmission via blood or blood product transfusion in most developed countries, perinatal or vertical transmission accounts for nearly all incident HIV infection in prepubertal children. HIV can be transmitted from mothers to infants during pregnancy through transplacental passage of the virus, presumably during labor and delivery through exposure to infected maternal blood and vaginal secretions, and during the postpartum period through breast-feeding. In utero transmission has been documented by identification of HIV in fetal tissue as early as 15 weeks,[2] although the exact timing of transmission during gestation is unknown.

The lack of a specific/sensitive diagnostic test for detection of HIV infection at birth has hindered our ability to document intrapartum transmission, which is presumed to occur similarly to hepatitis B virus transmission. Several cases of transmission to infants through breast-feeding by HIV-infected mothers have been documented in mothers who seroconverted while breast-feeding their infants[3,4]; HIV has also been isolated from cell-free breast milk.[5] Whether breast-feeding by mothers who were infected during pregnancy contributes significantly to transmission to infants who escaped in utero and intrapartum transmission is controversial; data from several studies are conflicting.[6–8]

Although the rate of transmission from mothers to infants varies from study to study, the larger, multicenter prospective studies report rates of about 25–35%.[6,7,9] with the exception of the European collaborative study which recently reported a rate of below 20%.[8] One study found that mothers with lower CD4 counts, below 400 cells/mm^3, and more advanced stage of disease were more likely to transmit HIV,[9] but other studies have not confirmed this relationship.[10] Three recent studies have found lower transmission rates in infants born to mothers with antibody to certain epitopes of the V3 loop of gp120 compared with infants born to mothers without these antibodies.[11–13] but other studies have been unable to confirm this finding.[14] Further study is clearly needed to examine factors that both promote and inhibit perinatal transmission.

The epidemiologic characteristics of children with perinatally acquired HIV infection reflect characteristics of women with the infection. HIV infection in women is largely associated with intravenous (IV) drug use or sexual contact with men who use drugs intravenously.[15] Rates of HIV infection among IV drug users have been highest in the northeastern states, particularly New York and New Jersey.[16] A disproportionate number of IV drug users in these areas are black or Hispanic. Thus most children with perinatally acquired infection reside in these areas and are black or Hispanic. As the epidemic spreads to other areas of the country, the demographic characteristics of the women and children will differ depending on the characteristics of the drug-using population in that area.

Transfusion and Hemophilia-Associated Transmission

Transfusion of HIV-infected blood or blood products is the most efficient means of HIV transmission. Studies have shown that more than 95% of persons receiving an HIV-seropositive transfusion have become infected.[17] One study also found shorter incubation/latency periods to development of AIDS in persons receiving blood/blood products from donors who developed AIDS soon after donation compared with persons receiving transfusions from donors in the earlier stages of the disease.[18]

The epidemiologic characteristics of children with transfusion-associated AIDS reflect the population of children being transfused. Most cases have occurred in children who received transfusions in the newborn period for perinatal conditions.[19] Cases have also occurred in children with congenital anemia (sickle cell, thalasemia) and other conditions requiring multiple transfusions. Thus, most cases to date have been infants and toddlers reflecting a mean incubation period of less than 5 years.[19] While most children are white (54%), a disproportionate number of children have been black (22%) or Hispanic (22%), probably because of the higher prevalence of low birth weight and other perinatal problems that place these children at greater risk of receiving blood/blood product transfusions. The geographic distribution of pediatric transfusion-associated AIDS cases within the United States reflects the seroprevalence in donor populations before donor screening. More than half (61%) of the cases have been from California, New York, New Jersey, Florida, or Texas.[19]

Children with coagulation disorders who received clotting factor between 1978 and 1985 were at particularly high risk of HIV infection. As many as 80% of children receiving large-pool, nonheat-treated factor products from plasma donated before HIV screening have developed HIV infection.[20] More severe hemophilia and greater factor usage have been associated with a greater risk of HIV infection.[20] While some investigators have speculated that some hemophiliacs may have become "immunized" through receipt of virus inactivated during the factor separation process, studies have shown that virus can be isolated from virtually all HIV-seropositive hemophiliacs.[21]

The epidemiologic characteristics of children with hemophilia-associated HIV infection are more reflective of the general U.S. population: 70% are white, 13% are black, 13% are Hispanic, and 3% are of other races or ethnicity. Geographically, these cases are dispersed throughout the United States (CDC national AIDS surveillance).

Measures to control transmission of HIV through blood/blood products have virtually eliminated this form of transmission. Although blood donations from newly infected persons donating during the "window" period between initial infection and seroconversion would not be eliminated by antibody screening, studies estimate that the risk of acquiring HIV from screened blood/blood products is from 1 in 38,000 to 1 in 153,000.[22,23] AIDS cases, however, are continuing to occur in persons who received blood/blood products before donor screening because of the long incubation period for the disease (median for adults, 7–8 years; median for children, 3–5 years).[19]

Clinical Features of HIV Disease in Children

The pathophysiology of HIV infection in children is similar to that in adults, but there are important differences in the disease manifestations. Although *Pneumocystis carinii* pneumonia (PCP) is the most common opportunistic infection in both children and adults, another pulmonary condition, lymphoid interstitial pneumonitis, occurs in many pediatric cases but is very rare in adults. Recurrent bacterial infections have been reported more commonly in children.[24] Neurologic disease resulting in dementia in adults is more likely to cause developmental delay or loss of developmental milestones in young children. Weight loss and wasting in adults may appear as failure to thrive in children. Immunologic parameters may also differ. While normal standards for CD4 counts have not been well established for children, counts are higher than those seen in adults particularly for children under one year of age.[25]

In general, the incubation/latency period for AIDS is much shorter in children compared with adults.[19] Children acquiring HIV from their mothers or from blood transfusions given during the first year of life have the shortest median incubation period, less than 5 years. In fact, most children with perinatally acquired infection develop signs and symptoms of disease in the first year of life. Median incubation periods in adults have generally ranged from 7 to 10 years, and adults rarely develop signs or symptoms of the disease in the first 3 years after infection.[26]

Laboratory Diagnosis of HIV Infection in Children

Antibody to HIV

Enzyme Immunoassay and Western Blot

As in adults, tests for antibody to HIV are the primary means of laboratory diagnosis of HIV infection in children acquiring the virus through nonperinatal routes (i.e., transfusion/hemophilia-associated infection). Children with perinatally acquired infection, however, present unique problems. Because maternal IgG antibody to HIV is passed transplacentally to virtually all infants born to HIV-seropositive women, the presence of antibody in the infant does not necessarily indicate virus infection. Studies have shown that about 25–35% of infants born to infected women acquire HIV infection, while nearly 100% will test positive by enzyme immunoassay (EIA) or western blot in the neonatal period (0–28 days of life), and maternal antibody can persist for as long as 15–18 months of age (median age at seroreversion is about 10 months).[27] The standard (EIAs) and western blot (see Chapter 5) most efficiently detect IgG and cannot differentiate between maternal- and infant-derived antibody.

Several approaches have been suggested to overcome this problem. One of the simplest approaches is to look for new bands on serial western blots on samples taken in the first year of life. New bands indicate antibody production by the infant and thus infection, but these may not be observed in the majority of infected infants and may not appear until several months of age.[28] In one study, two of eight HIV-infected infants followed prospectively developed new bands on western blot.[28]

Another approach that has been used in other congenital infections is to monitor antibody titer. A rising titer indicates antibody production by the infant and thus infection, while a falling titer would indicate noninfection. While theoretically applicable to HIV, studies have shown that antibody titer as measured by the optical density reading of the EIA is not always correlated with the infection status of the infants.[28]

HIV-Specific IgA and IgM Assays

A more promising approach is to test for HIV-specific antibodies that do not cross the placenta, such as IgM or IgA (see Chapter 5). Recent studies have shown that assays for HIV-specific IgA may be useful in diagnosing perinatally infected infants. Using a panel of seroconversion samples tested for HIV-specific IgG, IgA, and IgM, Weiblen et al.[29] found that IgA appeared as early as IgG, but persisted longer than IgM, reacted with more protein bands, and showed more intense staining that IgM. Applying these assays to samples from infected infants, Weiblen et al.[30] found HIV-specific IgA antibodies in 23 of 23 samples from infected infants older than 12 months, 12 of 18 samples from infants 6–12 months of age, 5 of 10 samples from infants 3–5 months of age, and 2 of 13 samples from infants less than 3 months of age. IgA antibodies were present in twice as many samples as IgM. Although this test was only able to identify a small percentage of infants less than 3 months of age, it does appear to be a useful test for diagnosing somewhat older infants less than 1 year of age.

Assays for IgM have been less useful. One study found that results of HIV-specific IgM antibody tests did not correlate with cord blood cultures or the presence of signs and symptoms of AIDS in infants during the first year of life.[31] In another study, only four of eight HIV-infected infants had detectable anti-HIV IgM antibody.[28] These problems with the IgM assay could result from the interference in the assays used in these studies from abundant IgG, which can produce spurious results. Removal of IgG using protein G before performing the IgM or IgA assay, as was done by Weiblen et al. in the studies cited here,[29,30] appears to be important for improving the sensitivity and specificity of these assays.[29] In addition, further information is needed regarding the timing and levels of production of these antibodies in infants infected perinatally.

Importance of Clinical Follow-Up

The standard EIA and western blot alone cannot identify infected infants, but the use of these tests serially during the first 2 years of life, coupled with careful medical follow-up, is the most readily available and accurate method for definitive diagnosis. Infants who develop CDC-defined AIDS, those with milder signs and symptoms of HIV disease who have the classic immune abnormalities, and those with persistent antibody beyond 15–18 months of age regardless of symptoms are considered infected.[32] These definitions are outlined in more detail in the CDC Classification System for HIV in children under 13 years of age.[32]

Infants who remain well and lose maternal antibody are considered uninfected, although a few cases of virus-positive/antibody-negative children have been reported.[7,8] In some cases, children who became antibody negative later seroconverted to antibody positive.[28,33] While such cases have been reported, this phenomenon is thought to be rare.

p24 Antigen

In general, assays for p24 antigen have not been useful in diagnosing HIV infection during the time period after seroconversion and before the development of severe disease (asymptomatic phase). The abundant antibody to HIV that is usually present during this time period complexes with noncell-associated viral antigens preventing the antigens from reacting with the test reagents. As the disease progresses and signs and symptoms develop, antibody to p24 wanes and free p24 antigen increases in the plasma fraction, and the test may become positive. Studies have shown that p24 antigen is usually negative until late in the course of the disease in infants born to HIV-infected mothers because of the presence of maternal antibody.[27,34]

Despite the assay's very limited use for early diagnosis, it can be quite helpful in certain clinical settings where virus is present but antibody is at low levels or absent. p24 antigen is likely to be positive in persons (other than perinatally infected infants) in the "window" period after initial infection and before seroconversion, about 6–12 weeks in most persons.[22] Likewise, the p24 antigen assay may be positive in some infants who are hypogammaglobulinemic and do not produce antibody.[35] p24 antigen levels have also been useful in monitoring the effect of antiviral therapy[36] and as a prognostic marker for progression to AIDS.[37] This assay is also widely used to monitor HIV cultures.[38]

HIV Culture

The presence of a positive virus culture is definitive evidence of HIV infection, but its use as a diagnostic test is limited, particularly in the pediatric population. Cultures typically can take as long as 4–6 weeks to complete and thus are not necessarily a rapid means of diagnosis. Cultures are also costly and labor intensive and require special biosafety precautions to prevent exposure of laboratory personnel. Thus cultures have been more useful in the research setting than in the clinical diagnostic setting.

$CD4^+$ Cell Counts and PCP among HIV-Infected Children

Recent progress has been made in the use of $CD4^+$ cell counts as an indication for PCP prophylaxis in children. Although normal $CD4^+$ cell values in infants and young children at various ages have not been well established, existing data indicate that median values for HIV uninfected and infected children, especially infants, are significantly higher compared with values for adults.[25]. Normal median $CD4^+$ cell counts were 3,200/mm^3 during the first 6 months of life with a progressive decline to 2,600/mm^3 between 13 to 24 months of age, and to 1,700/mm^3 by 2 to 6 years of age. $CD4^+$ cell counts in perinatally infected infants with PCP diagnosed at less than 1 year of age demonstrated that 73% had $CD4^+$ cell counts <1,000/mm^3 and 90% had counts <1,500/mm.[25] This compares with HIV-infected adults where $CD4^+$ cell counts of <200/mm^3 are highly predictive of increased risk for PCP. Thus, the $CD4^+$ cell count clinically useful for identifying young children at risk for PCP or other AIDS complications is likely to be higher than that for HIV-infected adults.

Recent guidelines[25] recommend PCP prophylaxis for children based on age-related $CD4^+$ cell counts as follows: <1,500/mm^3 for children 1–11 months, <750/mm^3 for children 12–23 months, <500/mm^3 for children 24 months through 5 years, and <200/mm^3 for children 6 years and older. A $CD4^+$ percentage of less than or equal to 20%, or a prior episode of PCP, should be used a indication for prophylaxis regardless of the absolute count. Because of the early onset of PCP (frequently below 6 months of age) and the high mortality from the first episode, prophylaxis usually needs to be initiated in the first few months of life, often before definitive diagnosis of HIV infection is made.

Newer Diagnostic Techniques under Development

Polymerase Chain Reaction

Polymerase chain reaction (PCR) is a relatively recent technique that appears to be quite promising for early diagnosis and possibly prognosis of HIV infection in infants born to HIV-infected women.[27] Because this test detects proviral DNA, it avoids the problem of maternal antibody. The amplification process makes the test quite sensitive and specific if contamination can be avoided.[39] One study of serial samples collected from infants followed during the first 2 years of life found that approximately 50–60% of HIV-infected infants were PCR positive during the neonatal period (0–28 days of age), and virtually 100% were positive at some time during the postneonatal period.[27] Most infants were PCR positive by 6 months of age. Infants who developed AIDS during the first 18 months of life were more likely to be PCR positive in the neonatal period compared with infected infants who had milder couses. Other studies have found similar results when testing infants during the postneonatal period, but few have tested significant numbers of infants in the neonatal period.[40,41]

There are two possible explanations why infected infants may be negative in the neonatal period. Infected infants may be PCR negative in the neonatal period if transmission occurred late in gestation or during labor and delivery. Alternatively, transmission could have taken place in utero although the level of proviral DNA in newborn blood at birth is below the level detectable by the procedure.

PCR is also useful in documenting noninfection in infants who lose maternal antibody. In a study of 119 infants who lost maternal antibody, none had conclusive evidence of HIV infection by PCR.[42] Six of the 119 infants tested PCR positive on one occasion, but none could be confirmed by repeat PCR testing or other laboratory or clinical examination. The authors suspected that the single positive PCR tests were false-positive results caused by shipping, handling, or laboratory errors. In fact, HLA typing of discordant samples from the 6 children indicated mislabeling in at least 2 because the discordants' samples had different HLA types. Alternatively, these children could be truly infected with levels of virus below the limits of the test in most blood samples.

Several advantages of PCR further highlight its use as an early and rapid diagnostic test for newborns. The test can be done on 2–3 ml of blood, a volume that is practical to obtain from a newborn. The technique can be done in 1 day's time and is less biohazardous than HIV culture. Although the technique is not widely available, and quality assurance programs are lacking, the usefulness of this technique in many other settings should drive the technology towards a more simpler, routine test in the future. The limitations of this technique mainly relate to the problems of possible contamination, which have been described in another chapter (see Chapter 7).

In Vitro Antibody Production Assays

Another promising technique for diagnosis of perinatally infected infants is the in vitro antibody production assay. This technique measures antibody-producing cells rather than the antibody itself; the presence of these cells indicates stimulation by viral infection. There have been two primary methods of identifying these cells. In one method, carefully washed infant peripheral blood mononuclear (PBMC) cells stimulated with either pokeweed mitogen or Epstein–Barr (EB) virus are cultured. Culture supernatants are tested for antibody with standard methods. Amadori et al.[43] detected spontaneously (unstimulated) antibody-secreting cells in 9 of 16 infected infants using EIA as the detection method and 14 of 16 using western blot. The use of pokeweed mitogen did not appear to improve the assay. Using Epstein–Barr stimulation, Pawha et al.[44] found HIV antibody-secreting cells in 23 of 24 (96%) symptomatic infected infants. Spontaneous antibody production was present in 10 of 24 (42%), and 17 of 24 (71%) were positive in pokeweed mitogen-stimulated cultures. The specificity of the assays in both studies was 100%.

In the second method, called ELISPOT, carefully washed infant PBMC are placed in wells with nitrocellulose membrane bottoms coated with HIV antigen (Figures 11.1 and 11.2). The cells are incubated, washed, then treated sequentially with biotinylated antihuman IgG, horseradish-conjugated avidin, and enzyme substrate. The appearance of "spots" on the nitrocellulose membrane indicates the presence of HIV-specific antibody-producing cells in the patient. Using this method, Lee et al.[45] detected HIV antibody-producing cells in 15 of 21 (72%) children with symptomatic infection. The antigen used to coat the wells may affect the sensitivity of the assay. Lee et al. used a recombinant peptide containing 82 amino acid residues encoded by a gene segment in the *env* region (gp41). The use of additional antigens might improve the sensitivity.

To summarize the studies, this method of diagnosis appears to be highly specific, and sensitivity ranges from 56% (unstimulated cells, using EIA as detection method) to 96% (E–B virus-stimulated cells). From data on adults presented in two of the three studies just described, sensitivity appeared to be somewhat lower in asymptomatic vs symptomatic individuals.

These assays are quite promising but have some important limitations. Studies to date have not tested large numbers of specimens collected in the neonatal period, a time when circulating maternal B cells could be present and cause false-positive results. Additionally, in the presence of abundant maternal IgG, false-positive tests may result from detection (in

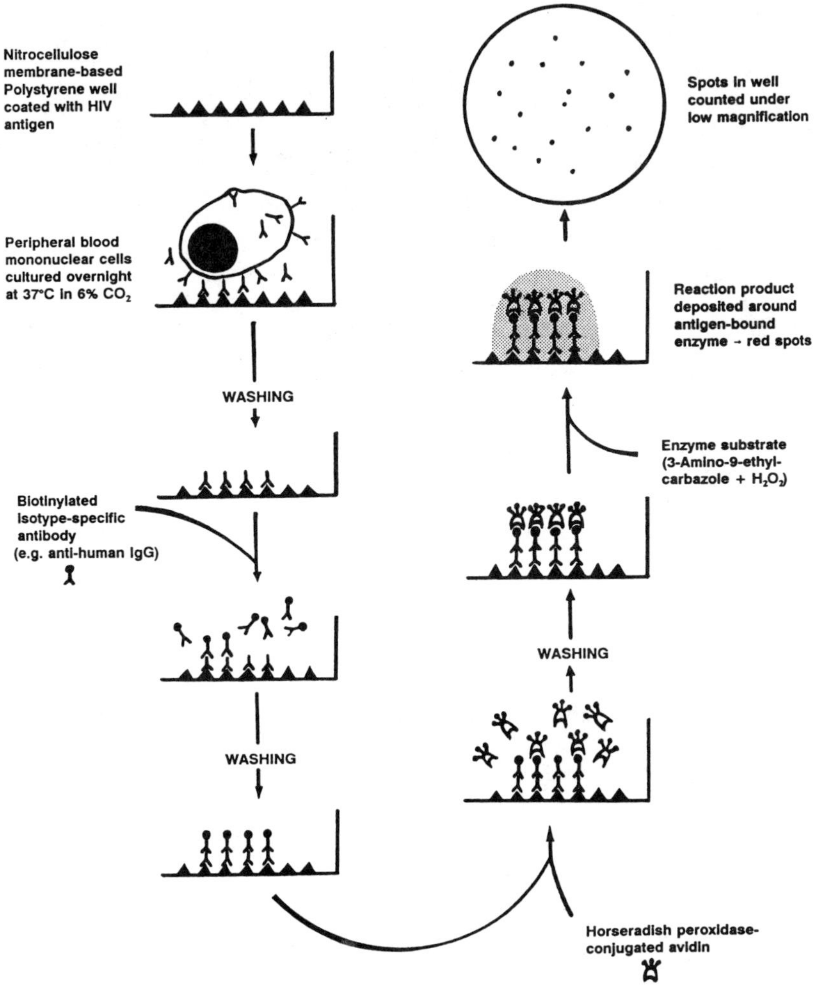

FIGURE 11.1. Schematic of ELISPOT assay for HIV-specific antibody-secreting cells. Washed peripheral blood mononuclear cells (PBMCs) are placed in wells with nitrocellulose membrane bottoms coated with HIV antigen. Cells are incubated, washed, then treated sequentially with biotinylated antihuman IgG, horseradish-conjugated avidin, and enzyme substrate. Appearance of "spots" on the nitrocellulose membrane indicates presence of HIV-specific antibody-producing lymphocytes in the patient.

culture supernates) of maternal anti-HIV antibody that has adhered to B cells from uninfected infants.[46] The ELISPOT method may be better able to differentiate between this carryover and true HIV antibody producing-cells.[47] The adsorbed antibody will yield a diffuse pink background stain-

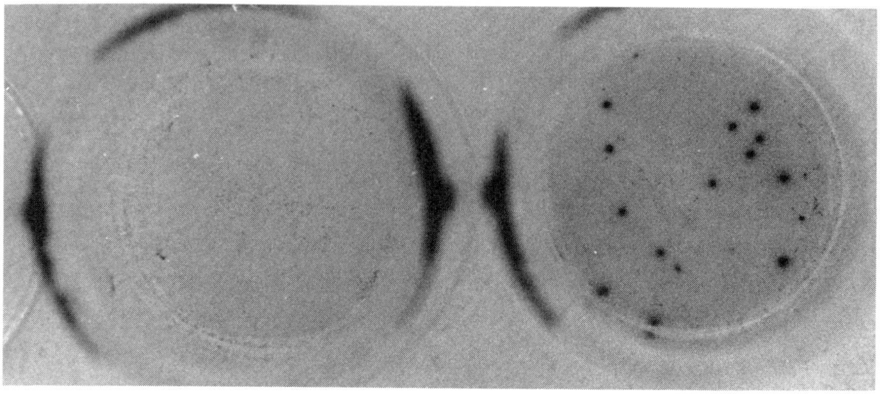

FIGURE 11.2. ELISPOT assay. Well on left represents incubation with peripheral blood mononuclear cells (PBMCs) from uninfected person; well on right represents incubation with PBMCs from HIV-infected person. Dark spots represent secretion of HIV-specific antibodies from infected person's PBMCs.

ing that can be readily distinguished from the intense red spots resulting from true antibody-producing cells.

Antibody secretion and the number of antibody-secreting cells might be influenced by treatment with zidovudine (AZT), thus affecting the sensitivity of these tests. Lee et al.[45] found that 12 of 16 (75%) of untreated adults were ELISPOT positive, while only 1 of 13 (8%) of AZT-treated adults were positive. Pawha et al.[44] found only transient changes in results from patients tested during the course of AZT therapy.

In vitro antibody production assays would not identify infected persons who are not producing antibody, such as hypo/agammaglobulinemic persons or possibly those with latent infection with absent or low viral replication. Active viral replication serves as the stimulus for replication of antibody-producing cells. Thus, in vitro antibody production assays may have a lower sensitivity for conditions associated with low levels of viral replication (i.e., AZT therapy or latent/asymptomatic stage of disease).

Synthesis of Results from All Assays

Despite the problems of early infant diagnosis, newer assays and improvements of older techniques are quite promising. Clinicians no longer need to wait until 15–18 months of age to make a definitive diagnosis. Most assays, including PCR, in vitro antibody production, HIV-specific IgA, and virus culture, have fairly high sensitivities (75–100%) by 6 months of age. Newborn/neonatal diagnosis however, remains a problem in that both PCR[27] and culture[48] detect only approximately 50% of infected infants during this time period. HIV-specific IgA[30] and p24 antigen assays[34] detect less than 10% of infants in the neonatal period. In vitro antibody production assays do not appear to be reliable during the first 1–2 months of life.[46] Very few neonatal samples have been tested using the ELISPOT method, but preliminary results appear promising.[47] Further studies are needed of samples from infants aged 1–6 months to determine the earliest age at which these tests are reliable for diagnosis.

While these tests are available to a varying extent in research, they are not widely available outside these settings. Standardization of methods and quality assurance programs also are not in place for these assays. With the exception of the p24 antigen assay, none of these assays are licensed by the U.S. Food and Drug Administration. PCR may soon be available in kit form but must undergo extensive evaluation before licensure. At present, clinicians usually accept two or more positive results on sequentially collected samples, particularly if confirmed by more than one assay method from those labs with a proven "track record" that have optimized their assay and are including proper laboratory controls.

Evaluation of Newer Tests

Continued evaluation of PCR, in vitro antibody production assays, HIV-specific IgA, and other diagnostic tests for early diagnosis of HIV infection in infants is critically needed. Therapies aimed at prevention and intervention are presumably most effective if given as early in the course as possible. To avoid possible complications of therapy in uninfected infants who would derive no benefit from the therapy, a sensitive and specific diagnostic test for newborns is needed.

In our haste to develop these techniques, however, several important factors should be kept in mind. First, the level of circulating virus and the percentage of infected cells changes throughout the course of the disease.[49,50] In addition, the timing of viral transmission from the mother to the infant is unknown. Thus, neonatal specimens should be analyzed separately from postneonatal specimens, and results from specimens taken from asymptomatic persons are not comparable to results from specimens taken from symptomatic persons. Studies that attempt to evaluate diagnostic techniques must report the age of the children at testing and the clinical stage of disease for the results to be interpretable and comparable to other studies.

Second, there is no single test that is sufficiently sensitive, specific, and standardized that it can serve as a "gold" standard. Careful clinical follow-up to at least 15–18 months is needed. Extreme caution should be used in interpreting a single diagnostic test, both for diagnosis and research. The emotional trauma caused by a wrong diagnosis and the damage caused by unsound public health policy based on uncomfirmed data is substantial.

References

1. CDC. Update: acquired immunodeficiency syndrome: United States, 1989. MMWR 1990;39:81–86.
2. Sprecher S, Soumenkoff G, Puissant F, Degueldre M. Vertical transmission of HIV in a 15-week fetus. Lancet 1986;2:288–289.
3. Oxtoby MO. Human immunodeficiency virus and other viruses in human milk: placing the issues in broader perspective. Pediatr Infect Dis J 1988;7: 825–835.
4. Hira SK, Mangrola UG, Mwale C, Chintu C, Tembo G, Brady WE, Perine PL. Apparant vertical transmission of human immunodeficiency virus type 1 by breast-feeding in Zambia. Journal of Pediatrics 1990;117:421–424.
5. Thiry L, Sprecher-Goldberger S, Jonckheer T, Levy J, Van de Perre P, Henrivaux P, Cogniaux-LeClerc J, Clumeck N. Isolation of AIDS virus from cell-free breast milk of three healthy virus carriers. Lancet 1985;ii: 891–892.
6. Blanche S, Rouzioux C, Moscato MG, Veber F, Mayaux M-J, Jacomet C, et al. A prospective study of infants born to women seropositive for human immunodeficiency virus type 1. N Engl J Med 1989;320:1643–1648.
7. Italian Mulicentre Study. Epidemiology, clinical features, and prognostic factors of pediatric HIV infection. Lancet 1988;ii:1043–1045.
8. The European Collaborative Study. Children born to women with HIV-1-infection: Natural history and risk of transmission. Lancet 1991;337:253–260.
9. Ryder RW, Nsa W, Hassig SE, Behets F, Rayfield M, Ekungola B, et al. Perinatal transmission of the human immunodeficiency virus type 1 to infants of seropositive women in Zaire. N Engl J Med 1989;320:1637–1642.
10. Thomas PA, NYC Perinatal HIV Transmission Collaborative Study Group. Early predictors and rate of perinatal HIV disese. In: abstracts, Vth International Conference on AIDS, Montreal, Canada, 1989.
11. Goedert JJ, Mendez H, Drummond JE, et al. Mother-to-infant transmission of human immunodeficiency virus type 1: association with prematurity or low anti-gp 120. Lancet 1989;ii:1352–1354.
12. Rossi P, Moschese V, Broliden PA, et al. Presence of maternal antibodies to human immunodeficiency virus 1 envelope glycoprotein gp 120 epitopes correlates with the uninfected status of children born to seropositive mothers. Proc Natl Acad Sci USA 1989;86:8055–8058.
13. Devash Y, Calvelli TA, Wood DG, Reagan KJ, Rubinstein A. Vertical transmission of human immunodeficiency virus is correlated with the absence of high affinity/avidity maternal antibodies to the gp120 principal neutralizing domain. Proc Natl Acad Sci USA 1990;87:3445–3449.
14. Shaffer N, Parekh BS, Pau CP, Abrams E, Thomas P, Krasinski K, et al. and the NYC Perinatal HIV Transmission Collaborative Study. Maternal antibodies to V3 loop peptides of gp120 are not associated with lack of perinatal HIV-1 transmission. In: VII International Conference on AIDS, Abstract # WC48. Florence, Italy, June 1991.
15. Oxtoby MJ. Perinatally aquired human immunodeficiency virus infection. Pediatr Infect Dis J 1990;9:609–619.

16. Hahn RA, Onorato IM, Jones TS, Dougherty J. Prevalence of HIV infection among intravenous drug users in the United States. JAMA 1989;261: 2677–2684.
17. Ward JW, Deppe DA, Samson S, et al. Risk of human immunodeficiency virus infection from blood donors who later developed the acquired immunodeficiency syndrome. Ann Intern Med 1987;106:61–62.
18. Ward JW, Bush TJ, Perkins HA, Lieb LE, Allen JR, Goldfinger D, et al. The natural history of transfusion-associated infection with human immunodeficiency virus. N Engl J Med 1989;321:947–952.
19. Jones DJ, Byers R, Bush T, Rogers MF. The epidemiology of transfusion-associated AIDS in children in the United States, 1981–1988. Pediatrics (in press).
20. Jason J, McDougal S, Holman CR, et al. Human T-lymphotropic retrovirus type III/lymphadenopathy-associated virus antibody. JAMA 1985;253: 3409–3415.
21. Jackson JB, Sannerud KJ, Hopsicker JS, Kwok SY, Edson JR, Balfour HH. Hemophiliacs with HIV antibody are actively infected. JAMA 1988;260: 2236–2239.
22. Ward JW, Holmberg SD, Allen JR, Cohn DL, Critchley SE, Kleinman SN, et al. Transmission of human immunodeficiency virus (HIV) by blood transfusions screened as negative for HIV antibody. N Engl J Med 1988;318: 473–478.
23. Cohen ND, Muñoz A, Reitz BA, Ness PK, Frazier OH, Yawn DH, et al. Transmission of retroviruses by transfusion of screened blood in patients undergoing cardiac surgery. N Engl J Med 1989;320:1172–1176.
24. Bernstein LJ, Krieger BZ, Novick B, Sicklick MJ, Rubinstein A. Bacterial infection in the acquired immune deficiency syndrome of children. Pediatr Infect Dis J 1985;4:472–475.
25. CDC. Guidelines for prophylaxis against *Pneumocystis carinii* pneumonia for children infected with human immunodeficiency virus. MMWR 1991;40: 1–13.
26. Hessol NA, Lifson AR, O'Malley PM, Doll LS, Jaffe HW, Rutherford GW. Prevalence, incidence, and progression of human immunodeficiency virus infection in homosexual and bisexual men in hepatitis B vaccine trials; 1978–1988. Am J Epidemiol 1989;130:1167–1175.
27. Rogers MF, Ou CY, Rayfield M, Thomas PA, Schoenbaum EE, Abrams E, et al. Use of the polymerase chain reaction for early detection of the proviral sequences of human immunodeficiency virus in infants born to seropositive mothers. N Engl J Med 1989;320:1649–1654.
28. Johnson JP, Nair P, Hines SE, Seiden SW, Alger L, Revie DR, et al. Natural history and serologic diagnosis of infants born to human immunodeficiency virus-infected women. Am J Dis Child 1989;143:1147–1153.
29. Weiblen BJ, Schumacher RT, Hoff R. Detection of IgM and IgA HIV antibodies after removal of IgG with recombinant protein G. J Immunol Methods 1990;126:199–204.
30. Weiblen BJ, Lee FK, Cooper ER, Landesman SH, McIntosh K, Harris JS, et al. Early diagnosis of HIV infection in infants by detection of IgA HIV antibodies. Lancet 1990;i:988–990.
31. Ryder RW, Hassig SE. The epidemiology of perinatal transmission of HIV. AIDS 1988;2:583–589.

32. Centers for Disease Control. Classification system for human immunodeficiency virus (HIV) infection in children under 13 years of age. MMWR 1987; 36:225–236.
33. Aiuti F, Luzi G, Mezzaroma I, Scano G, Papetti C. Delayed appearance of HIV infection in children. Lancet 1987;ii:858.
34. Borkowsky W, Krasinski K, Paul D, Holzman R, Moore T, Bebenroth D, et al. Human immunodeficiency virus type 1 antigenemia in children. J Pediatr 1989;114:940–945.
35. Borkowsky W, Krasinski K, Paul D, Moore T, Bebenroth D, Chandwani S. Human-immunodeficiency-virus infections in infants negative for anti-HIV by enzyme-linked immunoassay. Lancet 1987;i:1168–1171.
36. Chaisson RE, Allain J, Volberding PA. Significant changes in HIV antigen level in the serum of patients treated with azidothymidine. N Engl J Med 1986;315:1610–1611.
37. Fahey JL, Taylor JMG, Detels R, Hofmann B, Melmed R, Nishanian P, et al. The prognostic value of cellular and serologic markers in infection with human immunodeficiency virus type 1. N Engl J Med 1990;322:166–172.
38. Feorino PM, Forrester B, Schable C, Warfield D, Schochetman G. Comparison of antigen assay and reverse transcriptase assay for detecting human immunodeficiency virus in culture. J Clin Microbiol 1987;25:2344–2346.
39. Schochetman G, Ou CY, Jones WK. Polymerase chain reaction. J Infect Dis 1988;158:1154–1157.
40. Krivine A, Vakudima A, LeMay ML, Pena-Cruz V, Huang AS, McIntosh K. A comparative study of virus isolation, polymerase chain rection, and antigen detection in children of mothers infected with human immunodeficiency virus. J Pediatr 1990;116:372–376.
41. Chadwick EG, Yogev R, Kwok S, Sninsky JJ, Kellogg DE, Wolinsky SM. Enzymatic amplification of the human immunodeficiency virus in peripheral blood mononuclear cells from pediatric patients. J Infect Dis 1989;160: 954–959.
42. Abrams EA, Rogers MF, Ou C-Y, et al. Lack of HIV proviral sequences in children who have lost maternal antibody following birth to HIV (+) mothers. In: abstracts, VIth International Conference on AIDS, San Francisco, 1990.
43. Amadori A, De Rossi A, Giaquinto C, Faulkner-Valle G, Zacchello F, Chieco-Bianchi L. In-vitro production of HIV-specific antibody in children at risk of AIDS. Lancet 1988;i:852–854.
44. Pahwa S, Chirmule N, Leombruno C, Lim W, Harper R, Bhalla R, et al. In vitro synthesis of human immunodeficiency virus-specific antibodies in peripheral blood lymphocytes of infants. Proc Natl Acad Sci USA 1989;86:7532–7536.
45. Lee FK, Nahmias AJ, Lowery S, Nesheim S, Reef S, Thompson S, et al. ELISPOT: a new approach to studying the dynamics of virus-immune system interaction for diagnosis and monitoring of HIV infection. AIDS Res Hum Retrovir 1989;5:517–523.
46. De Rossi A. Antibody secreting cells (IVAP). In: Workshop on Early Diagnosis of HIV Infection in Infants, Washington, DC, 1990.
47. Lee F. Elispot. In: Workshop on Early Diagnosis of HIV Infection in Infants, Washington, DC, 1990.

48. Rousieux C. HIV culture in infants. In: Workshop on Early Diagnosis of HIV Infection in Infants, Washington, DC, 1990.
49. Ho DD, Moudgil T, Alam M. Quantitation of human immunodeficiency virus type 1 in the blood of infected persons. N Engl J Med 1989;321:1621–1625.
50. Coombs RW, Collier AC, Allain JP, Nikora B, Leuther M, Gjerset G, et al. Plasma viremia in human immunodeficiency virus infection. N Engl J Med 1989;321:1626–1631.

12 Other Human Retrovirus Infections: HTLV-I and HTLV-II

MICHAEL D. LAIRMORE and RENU LAL

The first human retrovirus described, human T-lymphotropic virus type 1 (HTLV-I), is considered the cause of adult T-cell leukemia/lymphoma.[1] More recently, the virus has been etiologically associated with tropical spastic paraparesis (TSP).[2] This chronic neurodegenerative disorder is clinicopathologically identical to HTLV-I-associated myelopathy (HAM), first described by Osame et al in Japan.[3] The list of HTLV-I-associated diseases may not be complete, because more clinical syndromes are being associated with the virus infection, exemplified by the recent descriptions of polymyositis and polyarthritis in HTLV-I-infected subjects.[4,5] Less clear are the disease associations, transmission routes, and epidemiologic features of HTLV-II infections. HTLV-II was initially isolated from a patient with hairy cell leukemia[6] and has subsequently been isolated only sporadically[7]; detailed studies of the pathogenesis of HTLV-II infection have not been reported. Recent studies using the polymerase chain reaction (PCR) technique have indicated that a high percentage of HTLV seroreactivity among intravenous (IV) drug users and blood donors in certain regions of the United States may be caused by HTLV-II.[8]

Serologic surveys of HTLV-I have provided important information regarding the distribution and disease associations of this retrovirus infection. The detection of antibodies remains a primary tool for epidemiologists interested in population-based studies of HTLV infection. The first and most widely used systems of antibody detection remain the enzyme-linked immunosorbent assays (ELISA), which have traditionally relied on whole virus preparations for their antigen preparations. Recent developments of recombinant and synthetic peptide-based immunoassay systems provide promise as more sensitive and specific assays for the diagnosis of HTLV infections. The verification of HTLV infection has also depended on virus isolation; tissue culture techniques have allowed the long-term culture of human lymphocytes and expression of the often transcriptionally inactive agent. The recent development of antigen capture systems to detect and quantitate small quantities of HTLV core antigens have increased the sensitivity and accuracy of HTLV culture systems.[9] In addition, the use of gene amplification (i.e., polymerase chain reaction) has revolutionalized the ability to detect HTLV proviral DNA and has allowed dramatic improvements in virus detection compared to the labor-intensive procedures of virus isolation.[10]

This chapter summarizes the biology and clinical features of HTLV-I and HTLV-II infection and disease. Through the knowledge of the virus replication strageties has come information regarding the potential pathogenic mechanisms of this group of retroviruses. Current serologic and virologic techniques to detect HTLV infection have greatly aided epidemiologic investigations for these viruses; these methods are described as a basis for understanding the often difficult task of human retrovirus discovery.

The Biology of HTLV Infection

The HTLV family shares structural features in common with all retroviruses, including the viral genes for group-specific antigens (*gag*), reverse transcriptase (*pol*), and envelope (*env*) proteins. However, HTLV-I and HTLV-II contain unique regulatory genes, which code for important transactivating proteins (e.g., *tax* and *rex*) at the 3′ end of the provirus (Table 12.1). These transacting proteins are analogous to the *tat* and *rev* proteins encoded by the human immunodeficiency virus (HIV); however, subtle differences exists in the mechanisms of transactivation between HTLV and HIV.

TABLE 12.1. Human T-lymphotropic virus type 1 genomic organization.

Gene	Function	protein product (kd)
Long terminal repeat (*ltr*)	Regulation	Non coding
Group-specific antigen (*gag*)	Core proteins	p53 precursor p19 matrix p24 capsid p15 nucleocapsid
Protease (*pro*)	*gag* cleavage	p14 protease
Polymerase (*pol*)	Replication	p62 transcriptase[a] p32 integrase[a]
Envelope (*env*)	Envelope	p61-68 precursor gp46 surface gp21 transmembrane
X Region (*pX*)	Regulation	p40x-*tax* (transactivation) p27/21x-*rex*

[a] Predicted protein product.

Retroviruses initiate their replication by binding to specific host cellular receptors through complementary viral envelope components. Unlike HIV, the cell receptor responsible for HTLV entry is not known. Somatic cell hybrid studies have suggested that the receptor for HTLV-I is associated with chromosome 17,[11] but further details of the receptor have not been reported. Following penetration of the host cell, single-stranded viral RNA with associated nucleoproteins and reverse transcriptase is released to allow synthesis of a DNA copy of the viral RNA. The resulting DNA copy (provirus) may either integrate into the host genome or remain extrachromosomal; it then initiates synthesis of viral RNA copies. Repeated nucleotide sequences (terminal repeat segments) at either end of the viral genome, in concert with viral and host genes, control viral replication. During productive phases of retrovirus replication, progeny virus bud from host cell membranes (often obtaining host proteins in the process) and are released to infect other cells. Transcriptional blocks of virus replications, defective viral genomes, and highly regulated viral encoded proteins allow some retroviruses to remain latent in the host cell genome.

Three mRNA species have been identified for HTLV: (i) a full-length genomic mRNA encoding for *gag* and *pol* proteins that is packaged in the virion; (ii) a 4.2-kilobase (kb) subgenomic mRNA with one intron removed through splicing that encodes the *env* protein; (iii) a 2.1-kb subgenomic mRNA, doubly spliced, that encodes for *tax* and *rex* proteins.[12] The *tax* reading frame produces a 40-kilodalton (kd) protein in HTLV-I and a 37-kd protein in HTLV-II; however, both proteins share similar features including localization in the nucleus of the infected cell. The *cis*-acting sequences that respond to *tax* are contained within a unique 3′ region (U3) of the long terminal repeat (LTR). Transactivation mediated by the tax protein in cooperation with host proteins may upregulate both virus LTR sequences and certain host genes. These activated genes include those that encode for the interleukin 2 receptor-alpha subunit (IL-2Ra), IL-2, certain oncogenes such as *c-fos*, and granulocyte-macrophage colony stimulating factor (GM-CSF).[13–15] This property of activation of cellular genes allows HTLV to overcome cellular controls and cause inappropriate expression of particular genes (e.g., host transcriptional factors), which may allow the eventual transformation of the cell. The role of the *tax* gene in carcinogenesis was supported by recent reports of mesenchymal tumors in mice transgenic for HTLV-I-*tax* gene,[16] the active expression of *tax* within lymphoma cells,[17] and transformation of cells transfected with plasmid vectors containing the *tax* gene.[18]

Like *tax*, the *rex* protein is localized in the nucleus, but is more specifically associated with the nucleoli where it appears to act after transcription to regulate the expression of viral genes.[12] Of the two proteins identified to be expressed by the *rex* open reading frame, p21 and p27, the larger protein p27 has been more extensively characterized.

The *rex* gene is required for the expression of incompletely spliced mRNA that encodes for the structural proteins of HTLV. The *rex* protein appears to increase the transport of unspliced *gag/pol* and singly spliced mRNA from the nucleus to the cytoplasm of infected cells; this process thus favors the production of viral structural proteins at the expense of the regulatory proteins.

The LTR of HTLV contain 21-bp repeat sequences that have nucleotide sequences in common with cyclic AMP- (c-AMP-) responsive elements.[19] Therefore, it is not unexpected that the HTLV-LTR has been demonstrated to respond to cAMP and other activators of cellular protein kinase C pathways. This responsiveness to host activation signals has important implications in understanding how the virus is regulated and how the state of the host cell determines the extent of viral replication.

The mechanism of the way in which HTLV causes adult T-cell leukemia is not completely understood. HTLV can induce cell proliferation by several mechanisms. The virion itself is mitogenic (e.g., envelope proteins) and can induce resting T lymphocytes to proliferate.[20] This exogenous proliferative effect may enhance the further replication of the virus. After HTLV begins to replicate, the *tax* gene product may induce proliferation (e.g., through the induction of IL-2Ra). This autocrine effect may cause the infected cell to be more susceptible to further signals of transformation.

The role of the virus in the case of HTLV-I-associated myelopathy is equally unclear. The virus is difficult to detect by conventional methods (in situ hybridization, immunofluorescence) at lesion sites with the spinal cord and brain. Therefore, a direct viral-mediated injury does not appear to explain the intense lymphocytic infiltrates demonstrated in the affected HAM/TSP patients.[21] Recent ultrastructural demonstration of $CD8^+$ lymphocytes intimately associated with degenerate myelinated nerve fibers of a HAM/TSP patient, in the absence of HTLV antigens, indicated that indirect cell-mediated damage may be operative in the induction of the lesion.[22] Demonstration of neural cell culture damage by the cerebrospinal fluid (CSF) of HAM/TSP patients may suggest that soluble mediators play a role in the myelin damage of HAM/TSP. The HTLV-I *tax* gene, when transfected into rat glial cell cultures, can induce class I major histocompatibility complex antigen expression, which could potentially allow glial cells to serve inappropriately as antigen-presenting cells.[23]

The predominant cell target of HTLV appears to be the $CD4^+$ lymphocyte. This lymphocyte subtype is the predominant tumor cell phenotype associated with adult T-cell leukemia/lymphoma (ATLL) cases[24] and is the predominant cell type demonstrated to be transformed in culture. In addition, recent PCR amplification of various leukocyte subtypes from HAM/TSP patients suggested that the $CD4^+$ lymphocyte population contained more than 90% of the viral sequences.[25] The association of HTLV with neurologic disease has created interest in identification of potential neural cell targets for the virus. In vitro rat glial cells have been demonstrated to support the replication of HTLV-I; however, the biological relevance of this observation is unclear because this cell type has not been demonstrated to be infected in human autopsy material. HTLV-I has been isolated from HAM/TSP patients' CSF cells and has been used to establish CSF-derived cells lines.[26] Thus far, no specific nucleotide sequence differences have been discovered that are unique to HAM/TSP isolates.[27] Thus, the pathogenesis of HTLV either in the induction of lymphoproliferative or neurologic disease is far from clear, and further research in this area is needed.

Clinical Aspects of HTLV Infection

Although HTLV-I has routes of transmission similar to those of HIV, HTLV-I is highly cell associated. This cell-associated nature appears to explain epidemiologic studies demonstrating that the virus is more readily transmitted from infected males to females, presumably via infected leukocytes in seminal fluids. Familial clustering of the virus infection has been demonstrated; seropositive rates may be threefold higher among healthy relatives compared to healthy blood donors.[28] Among female spouses of HTLV-I-positive males, as many as 60% may seroconvert to HTLV-I over a 10-year period.[29]

Animal models of HTLV-I infection have provided data to support the sexual transmission of the virus. Among Japanese macaques, which harbor the closely related virus simian T-lymphotropic virus type 1 (STLV-I), sexual transmission was documented as early as 8 weeks after exposure, and male-to-female transmission was the predominant pattern of transmission. The virus has been isolated from infected human and monkey semen, and human semen from a seropositive individual was used to successfully infect rabbits following intravenous injection.[30] Among infected monkeys, those with the greatest antibody titers were more likely to transmit the virus, suggesting that virus load may play a role in the infectivity of an individual.[31]

HTLV-I is transmitted from infected mothers to their offspring, primarily via breast milk. The virus has been isolated from breast milk, and breast milk can transmit the virus infection to both rabbits and monkeys.[32] Virus culture and PCR studies of cord blood samples suggest that HTLV-I is not transmitted in utero. Further evidence that breast-feeding is the predominant mode of transmission of the virus from a seropositive mother to children have been obtained from epidemiologic studies in endemic locations. In Japan, seropositive mothers who bottle-fed their offspring were found to virtually eliminate transmission to their children.[33]

Parenteral injection of infected blood is a common means of transmission of HTLV-I. Blood transfusion of unscreened blood has been associated with seropositivity among multiply transfused patients[34] and has more recently been associated with acute-onset HAM/TSP.[35] In November 1988, the U.S. Food and Drug Administration issued a recommendation that all blood donated for transfusion in the United States be screened for HTLV-I.[36] This recommendation was based, in part, on a preliminary report (sponsored by the American Red Cross) of a 0.025% seropositive rate among volunteer blood donors.[37] In blood, the virus is associated with the cellular fractions that account for virtually all the transmission of the infection. Plasma and blood factor components apparently do not transmit the infection.[38] Among individuals who receive whole blood or cellular portions of blood, seroconversion occurs in approximately 60% of transfused individuals within 4 to 8 weeks after blood transfusion. Parenteral exposure to the virus from needle-sharing is a predominant mode of transmission of the virus among drug abusers. Seropositive rates are elevated among IV drug users and IV-drug-using female prostitutes.[39] In addition, black or hispanic race is an independent risk factor for HTLV-I infection among drug users. Although health care workers do not appear at risk for HTLV infection, the risk of exposure to HTLV-I-infected blood may be greater among hospital workers in certain inner-city populations that have elevated seropositive rates.[40]

The pathogenesis of HTLV-I infection and disease is poorly understood, in part because of the long latent period between exposure and disease manifestations. There appears to be no preferred site of HTLV proviral integration, and the genomes of HTLVs do not contain typical oncogenes (e.g., *c-myc*). Proposed mechanisms of HTLV-I tumor induction include a multistep model in which randomly integrated HTLV-I induces cellular proliferation (e.g., *tax*-mediated transactivation) and subsequent "secondary" signals then allow for the emergence of lymphocyte clones.[12] The spectrum of lymphoproliferative disease associated with HTLV-I infection includes acute adult T-cell leukemia/lymphoma (ATLL), smoldering ATLL, cutaneous T-cell lymphoma, and, less often, B-cell lymphoma.[24] The HTLV genome may be transcriptionally inactive in tumor cells (e.g., methylated) or may be partially deleted. ATLL is predominantly manifested as an aggressive $CD4^+$ T-cell lymphoma that is refractory to conventional therapeutic protocols. Hypercalcemia and occasionally eosinophilia may occur as secondary sequelae to ATLL; these syndromes may be caused by tax-mediated transactivation of cellular lymphokines.[41] The incubation period of ATLL may be measured in years to decades.

In contrast to the neoplastic nature of ATLL, HAM/TSP is a chronic neurodegenerative disease predominantly of the spinal cord that is characterized by lymphocytic infiltrates and myelin degeneration.[21] This syndrome has been confused clinically with multiple sclerosis (MS) but is neuropathologically distinct from it.[28] HAM/TSP patients tend to have a slowly progressive clinical course marked by paraparesis, difficulty in maintaining gait, impotence, and bladder dysfunction (Table 12.2). HAM/

TABLE 12.2. Human T-lymphotropic virus diseases associations.

HTLV-I	
Strongly Associated Diseases	
Adult T-cell leukemia/ lymphoma (ATLL)	Aggressive mature T-cell malignancy, skin lesions, lymphadenopathy, hypercalcemia, lytic bone lesions. Develops in 1–4% of HTLV-I-infected persons after prolonged latency. Median survival 11 months.
Tropical spastic paraparesis/HTLV-I-associated myelopathy (TSP/HAM)	Slowly progressive myelopathy of pyramidal tracts. Extremity weakness, back pain, incontinence, spasticity. Develops in 1–4% of HTLV-I-infected persons after moderate to prolonged latency. Long-term survival (years).
Reported Diseses (not conclusively linked to HTLV-I infection)	
Polymyositis	Nonhereditary myopathy, muscle weakness, wasting, necrosis, lymphocytic infiltrates.
Polyarthritis	Chronic nonsuppurative arthritis.
Alveolitis	Lymphocytic interstitial alveolitis.
HTLV-II	
No clear disease associations. HTLV-II has been isolated from at least two cases of hairy cell leukemia (HCL), but many HCL are HTLV-II negative.	

TSP lesions are concentrated primarily within the thoracic spinal cord and consist of lymphocytic meningeal and perivascular infiltrates and prominant demyelination. Unlike multiple sclerosis, HAM/TSP is not associated with prominant plaque formation within the nervous tissue. The latent period of HAM/TSP may depend on several factors, including viral dose (multiply transfused patients), host genetic factors (HLA haplotypes), or virus strain (unique viral determinants of neural tropism). HAM/TSP patients exhibit intense antibody responses to the viral infection and intrathecal production of anti-HTLV-I antibodies.[42] In addition, spontaneous proliferation of lymphocytes from HAM/TSP patients suggests that these individuals have increased immunologic responsiveness to the infection.[43]

Serologic Testing for HTLV

The detection of antibodies to retrovirus infections has been traditionally used as a marker to indicate either latent or active infection of the host. A variety of techniques are available to detect the presence of antibodies to HTLV-I and HTLV-II; many of these methods are similar to tests used to detect antibodies to HIV. This section summarizes available techniques used for detection of antibodies to HTLV infection and comments on emerging methods to improve the sensitivity and specificity of serologically based tests for HTLV-I and HTLV-II.

Viral infections are generally countered by the host immune response, which includes both humoral (e.g., production of antibodies) and cell-mediated (e.g., cytotoxic lymphocytes) immune responses. Antibodies gainst various viral structural proteins are measured by a number of simple and sensitive tests including enzyme immunoabsorbant assays (EIA), immunoblot or western blot (IB), immunofluorescence assay (IFA), radioimmunoprecipitation assay (RIPA), and particle agglutination (PA) (Table 12.3). Although antibodies have been detected to nearly all HTLV gene products those antibodies usually measured in serologic assays correspond to *gag*-encoded proteins (p19, p24, p53) and *env*-encoded glycoproteins (pg46 and gp61/68).

The enzyme immunoabsorbent assay (EIA) has several major advantages including economy and simplicity of use; it is also sensitive in the detection of antibodies to whole viral antigens. EIAs are rapid colorimetric tests that can be partially automated and can easily test large numbers of samples; EIA is the method of choice for screening donated blood.[44] Samples of serum or plasma to be tested are added to the solid-phase microtiter plates, which have been coated with antigen (usually whole viral preparatons). After incubation, bound antibodies are detected by a form of antiimmunoglobulin–enzyme conjugate (e.g., peroxidase-conjugated antihuman immunoglobulin). This complex is treated with an enzyme–substrate reactant, and a chromogen is used to produce a color reaction detected with a spectrophotometer. Within certain techical limitations, the quantity of antibodies present is proportional to the optical

TABLE 12.3. Serologic tests for human T-lymphotropic virus type I.

Immunofluorescent assay (IFA)	Antibodies reacted with HTLV-infected cells. Good sensitivity, not specific for individual gene product reactivity.
Particle agglutination assay (PA)	Latex bead-based assay. Good sensitivity, not specific for individual gene product reactivity. Used primarily in Japan.
Western blot or immunoblot (IB)	Antibodies react with separated antigen in nitrocellulose or nylon strips. Good sensitivity and specificity. Requires definition of positive result because of potential false-positive bands.
Radioimmunoprecipitation assay (RIPA)	Radiolabeled HTLV-infected cell lysates reacted with serum and then precipitated with sepharose beads. Good sensitivity and specificity. Labor intensive and expensive.
Recombinant/synthetic protein assays	Good sensitivity and specificity. Potential to differentiate HTLV-I from HTLV-II infection.

density of the test well. The rate of false-negatives (sensitivity) and false-positives (specificity) is a major concern in any serologic assay including EIAs.

To aid in the interpretation of EIAs, confirmatory pathways have been suggested to confirm HTLV seropositivity (Table 12.4). A sample that tests reactive in an initial EIA may be retested; if the subsequent test is nonreactive the sample may be considered negative for HTLV antibodies. Such nonrepeatably reactive EIA test results are usually attributed to technical errors or high negative control test signals. If a sample is repetively reactive on testing the sample is intepreted as being "reactive" for antibodies to HTLV. Additional, more specific supplemental tests (e.g., western blot) should be used to confirm "reactive" EIA samples.[45] If HTLV antibodies are not detected by these more specific tests, then the sample should be considered false-positive for HTLV antibodies. Such test results may be the result of sera containing antibodies that recognize cellular components of viral antigen preparations (e.g., major histocompatibility complex class I antigens).

Other causes of false-positive EIA test results are factors that may influence the nonspecific adherence of immunoglobulins to the solid phase of the EIA plate, such as repeated freezing and thawing of the serum specimen, lipemic serum specimens, serum containing hemolyzed red blood cells, or excessive agglutinated "sticky" serum. False-positive tests results may also result from the cross-reactivity of antibodies to other retroviruses. HTLV-II shares approximately 60–65% nucleotide sequences with HTLV-I and is antigenically extensively cross-reactive with HTLV-I.[6,45] Because of the close structural similarity between HTLV-I and HTLV-II, whole virus-based antigen tests for HTLV-I often react to HTLV-II antibodies and do not allow discrimination between these two viral infections.

Antibody reactivity to individual gene products of HTLV are not visible using EIA; western blot tests allow the discrimination of antibody reactivity to particular HTLV proteins. Because of the ease of use and specificity

TABLE 12.4. Confirmation of HTLV-I serologic test results.

1. Screening of serum/plasma sample by EIA, IFA, or PA.
2. Samples negative; no further testing.
   Samples repeatively reactive; require further supplemental tests (e.g., western blot or RIPA).
3. After WB and RIPA:
   - Samples negative; considered **negative**, no further testing.
   - **Samples *gag* p24 and *env* gp46 (or gp61) reactive; positive.**[a]
   - Samples with viral reactivity, but without positive criteria; **indeterminate**, require further testing.

[a] Recommended criteria by the U.S. Public Health Service.

of reactivity, the western blot is a standard "confirmatory" assay following initial EIA screening. Variation of the western blot technique may be used by different laboratories, but the basic principles for the test are similar. The diagnostic criteria for a positive HTLV-I serologic test have been recommended by a U.S. Public Health Service working group to include reactivity to both p24 and gp46 or gp61/68.[36] These recommendations were based, in part on the dominant reactivity among known infected individuals and the dominant antigens represented within the format of the immunoblot test (Figure 12.1).[44,45] Recent development of recombinant-based envelope (p21e) antigen assays may be a useful adjunct in the confirmation of antibody against HTLV-I envelope and eliminate the need to perform RIPA (R. Lal, unpublished data).

Serum specimens may be identified that are "indeterminate" following EIA and western blot tests; these samples may be reactivity to a least one viral specific band yet not satisfy the criteria of a seropositive sample (e.g., p19 only or p19 and p28, p24 only).[45] Indeterminate serum samples may be caused by several factors including low antibody titers, early seroconversion to the viral infection, HTLV-II-infection or other unknown closely related retroviruses, or antibodies against cellular components sharing epitopes with HTLV. Certain monoclonal antibodies against HTLV-I p19 have been demonstrated to recognize unique cellular antigens (e.g., cortical thymocytes).[46] Such indeterminate samples may be further classified by testing by RIPA; this assay appears to be more sensitive for the detection of reactivity of HTLV antibodies against the viral envelope.

The radioimmunoprecipitation assay (RIPA) is primarily a research method to detect HTLV antibodies, in part because it is complex. Because the RIPA is labor intensive, requiring facilities to handle HTLV-infected cell cultures and radionucleotides, the assay has been used to only a limited extent in routine diagnostic testing. However, the RIPA if performed optimally is particularly useful to detect antibodies to HTLV envelope gene products (e.g., gp61/68),[45] but will also detect antibodies to HTLV *gag* p24, p53, and, to a limited extent, p19. The RIPA assay is particularly useful to classify serum specimens that may be reactive to p24 only.

One form of RIPA is performed by first labeling the amino acids of an HTLV-infected cell culture with radionucleotides such as ^{35}S methionine. The labeled cell culture is then disrupted and the labeled lysate is incubated with the serum sample to be tested; subsequent immunoprecipitation and autoradiographic steps detect the viral antibodies. As with the western blot test, strict adherence to the use of control serum (positive and negative) and clear detection of the molecular weights of viral bands (i.e., comparisons with molecular weight standards or reactivity with monoclonal antibodies to HTLV proteins) are necessary for accurate serologic results.

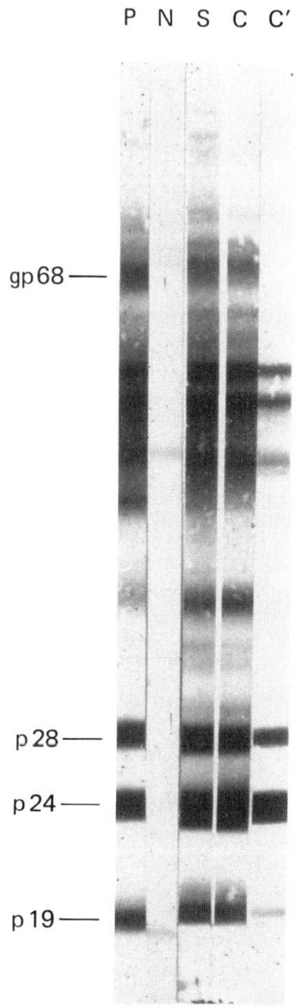

FIGURE 12.1. HTLV-I western blot assay. Nitrocellulose strips with HTLV-I antigen (MT-2 cell lysate) used to detect antibodies in HAM/TSP patient serum and cerebrospinal fluid (CSF). Lane P, positive control serum from adult T-cell leukemia/lymphoma (ATLL) patient. Lane N, negative control serum from normal donor. Lane S, 1:100 dilution of serum from HAM/TSP patient. Lane C, 1:10 dilution of CSF from HAM/TSP patient. Lane C′, 1:100 dilution of HAM/TSP patient serum. Antibody–antigen complexes detected by using peroxidase-labeled antihuman immunoglobulin and avidin–biotion complex assay. Molecular weight marks indicate location of major viral bands: gp68 envelope precusor and *gag* products p19, p24, and p28.

The immunofluorescence assay (IFA) has been a useful and technically simple assay employed to detect antibodies to retroviruses, including HTLV.[47] However, the IFA has not been as widely employed as immunoblot (IB), in part because the assay will not discriminate antibodies to particular gene products of HTLV. The primary advantage of the IFA is the convenience and rapidity with which test results may be obtained (approximately 30–60 minutes with directly conjugated IFA procedures). Like the EIA, the IFA test may allow for quantitation of antibodies and shares the potential problem of "false-positive" test results. In addition, the IFA is subjective in interpretation and requires considerable experience to properly interpret.

Although EIA test formats are convenient, the low positive predictive values of positive test results in typical infected populations limits their use as a single-step test procedure.[48] Recombinant protein-based or synthetic peptide-based assays offer attractive alternative methods for the screening of infected populations. These types of assays may be superior in screening because of the lack of cellular components within the antigen preparations and the noninfectious nature of the antigen production. These antigens may be "custom" designed to include antigens of particular usefulness in the serodiagnosis of HTLV infections or may be made to exclude certain peptide sequences homologous with host proteins.

The sensitivity of most western blot assays is limited in their ability to detect antibodies against HTLV-I envelope proteins; the sensitivity of these assays can be improved by "spiking" western blot strips with recombinant-derived HTLV-I envelope antigens.[49,50] One such recombinant protein has been employed to enhance both EIA and western blot assay detection of HTLV-I.[51] However, these assays remain cross-reactive for the detection of antibodies against HTLV-II infection. To increase the specificity of HTLV-I immunoassay, synthetic peptides derived from HTLV-I and HTLV-II amino acid sequences have been developed in several research laboratories. These assays derived from immunodominant epitopes offer potential alternative approaches to EIA-based tests.[52]

The use of synthetic or recombinant protein-based assays allows distinguishing the antibody reactivity against infection by HTLV-I from reactivity to HTLV-II infection. Certain domininant epitopes derived from HTLV-I or HTLV-II amino acid sequences have been demonstated to be useful in these assays to specifically determine antibodies against the viral infections in both research applications[52,53] and commercially available assays (e.g., Olympus Corporation, Lake Success, New York; Coulter Immunology, Hialeah, Florida).

Nucleic Acid Methods of Detection

The transcriptional activity of HTLV-I and HTLV-II within an infected host is highly regulated, and as a result the direct detection of viral proteins from cells or tissues is difficult. The integration of HTLV in the host cell genome is often followed by a transcriptional "block" (reduced expression of mRNA); this allows the virus to remain latent and cause lifelong infections. Therefore, methods used to detect viral nucleic acids have been employed to detect the presence of HTLV from infected cells.

Techniques to detect relatively large copy numbers of viral nucleic acid include both Southern blot assays and in situ hybridization. Each assay is dependent on the sensitivity and specificity of the probe used to detect proviral DNA, as well as the methods and tissues used in the preparations. In situ hybridization uses radiolabeled probes that consist of portions of the viral genome (e.g., single-stranded DNA) which are applied to specifically treated slides of cells or tissues.[54] This technique has the major advantage of morphologic identification of infected cells; however, it is technically difficult and less sensitive than gene amplification methods (e.g., polymerase chain reaction). Southern blot procedures are similar to in situ hybridization in preparation of labeled probes; however, the detection is based on identification of viral nucleic acids from blotted membranes. Restriction enzymes with unique cutting sites are used to allow predictions of the integration of HTLV from lymphoma cells or cell cultures. The ability of Southern blot to detect monoclonal integration of HTLV-I in tumor cells has been employed diagnostically to predict the status of ATLL patients.[55] Direct Southern blot of HTLV, like in situ hybridization, is technically difficult and is not sensitive to detect HTLV in low numbers of infected cells (e.g., seropositive but asymptomatic patients).

The application of polymerase chain reaction (PCR) for the detection of HTLV has allowed more sensitive and specific detection of this subfamily of retroviruses. The use of specific primers and probes have allowed investigators to discriminate the nucleic acids of HTLV-I from closely related retroviruses like HTLV-II.[10] This procedure is based on continuous cycles of amplification of a process of denaturing target DNA, annealing of primers, extension of the intervening segments with unique polymerase enzymes (i.e., *taq* polymerase), and finally detection of the specifically amplified target sequence.

The procedure has the major advantage of amplification of the viral signal (as much as a millionfold). However, because of the sensitivity of the assay, strict adherence to control procedures is necessary to avoid cross-contamination. Appropriate controls should include both negative and positive cell controls, molecular weight standards, sensitivity controls (serially diluted positive controls), and specificity controls (related but different viral cell lines). Controls and test samples should be prepared in the same manner to prevent variability in the methods of cell preparation. DNA for PCR can be prepared from cells simply by lysing in the presence of detergents or by using more rigorous methods of phenol extraction. Amplified products are detected after separation in agarose or acrylamide gels followed by transfer and probing by hybridization with labeled (e.g., ^{32}P) probes. Laboratory space used for all procedures involving DNA extraction should be separated physically from rooms used for amplification of the target DNA to prevent contamination of primer pairs and probes.

The development of PCR procedures for HTLV-I and HTLV-II have, for the first time, allowed investigations of the prevalence and potential disease associations of HTLV-II.[8] In addition, the use of PCR to directly diagnose individuals with HTLV infection has, in part, precluded the need to culture cells from these patients. Several important caveats must be kept in mind in the application of PCR to detect HTLV infection. The procedure detects the DNA of HTLV and does not provide information concerning the replication capacity or infectious nature of the virus infection. Because of potential cross-contamination problems and detection of endogenous retrovirus sequences, the criteria of a positive PCR test should include detection of HTLV from at least two separate portions of the genome (Table 12.5).

Culture Methods of HTLV

The detection of HTLV-I and HTLV-II by virus isolation is dependent on activation of T lymphocytes and cell culture conditions that allow for the long-term growth of lymphocytes. The viruses are transmitted by cell-to-cell transfer, and successful infections of cell cultures with cell-free virus preparations have generally been unsuccessful. Because of these biologic factors, virus isolation procedures require that test subjects' peripheral blood mononuclear cells (PBMC) or tumor material be stimulated (e.g., by mitogens) and monitored for the presence of viral reverse transcriptase, antigens, or nucleic acids. In addition, coculturing with appropriate uninfected target cells (e.g., mitogen-stimulated PBMC) will enhance the ability of detection of HTLV from infected persons. Mon-

TABLE 12.5. Diagnostic methods of detection of HTLV nucleic acids.

Methods	Procedure	Comments
Southern blot assay	DNA from HTLV cells blotted on membranes, reacted with labeled complimentary probes	Sensitivity determined by conditions of assay. Used to determine state of viral integration.
In situ hybridization	DNA or RNA in tissues reacted with labeled complimentary probes	Excellent to determine cellular location of infection. HTLV may be transcriptionally muted and RNA detection low.
Polymerase chain reaction (PCR)	DNA or RNA from HTLV cells reacted with primers, amplified enzymatically, and probed	Excellent sensitivity, can differentiate HTLV-I from HTLV-II; may result in false-positives.

itoring cultures for the presence of reverse transcriptase is often of limited value because of the low levels produced by this class of dretrovirus. In addition, the measurement of this retrovirus enzyme is not specific for HTLV and will also detect the presence of other retroviruses (e.g., HIV) and potentially detect endogenous host polymerases.

The development of sensitive (detection of as little as 0.1 ng/ml of core antigen) and specific (detection of HTLV-I specifically or both HTLV-I and HTLV-II) antigen capture assays has greatly improved the ability to detect HTLV from infected cell cultures.[7,9] These assays detect soluble antigens (primarily major core antigens) in cell culture supernatants using either polyclonal (rabbit anti-HTLV serum, Cellular Products, Buffalo, New York) or monoclonal (anti-p24 of HTLV-I/II, Coulter Immunology, Hialeah, Florida) antibodies to capture antigen. The bound antigen–antibody complex is detected colorimetrically. By comparison of the optical density readings of test samples with standard preparations, the quantitity of viral antigen within the culture can be estimated. Unlike the situation for HIV-infected persons, these HTLV antigen capture assays have not been universally employed to detect viral antigen directly from patients' bodily fluids (e.g., serum). This limitation of antigen detection from patients may be caused by several factors, including complexing of antigens with patients' antibodies or low levels of HTLV antigens due to the cell-associated nature of the viral infection. Alternate procedures to detect the presence of HTLV in cell cultures include IFA and avidin–biotin complex methods that allow visualization of viral antigens from the surface of infected cells (Table 12.6).

TABLE 12.6. Methods to detect HTLV antigens in cell culture.

Methods	Comments
Immunofluorescent assay	Simple to perform for detection of HTLV from infected cells. Cost effective, labile signal.
Avidin–biotin complex assay	Easily performed for detection of HTLV from infected cells. Stable signal; allows slide record.
p19 antigen capture assay[a]	Excellent specificity for HTLV-I antigen in cell culture supernatants. Will not detect HTLV-II antigen. Microtiter plate to test multiple samples.
p24 antigen capture assay[b]	Sensitive assay for HTLV-I and HTLV-II p24 antigen in cell culture supernatants. Microtiter plate to test multiple samples.

[a] p19 antigen capture assay (Cellular Products Company, Buffalo, New York).
[b] p24 antigen capture assay (Coulter Immunology, Hialeah, Florida).

Screening, Confirmation, and Counsel

The U.S. Public Health Service has published criteria for interpretation of HTLV-I serologic test results.[36] These criteria were based on the experiences of several references labortories and include the following recommendations: a serum specimen to be considered positive must have reactivity to both *gag* p24 and to an *env* gene product (gp46 or pg61/68); a serum specimen with no viral specific reactivity should be considered negative; and serum specimens not satisfying the seropositive criteria, but showing immunoreactivity to a least one suspected HTLV-I gene product, are designated "indeterminate." To establish the immunoreactivity of a serum specimen the sample may require testing by both western blot and RIPA. Samples that are reactive repeatedly in EIA but which contain no viral specific bands in western blot or RIPA should be considered negative. Most currently available serologic tests do not have the ability to distinguish between antibody reactivity to HTLV-I versus HTLV-II. To distinguish between patients with these infections, virus isolation, PCR, or serologic assays that are based upon synthetic peptides or recombinant proteins must be employed.

Blood donors whose serum samples are repeatably reactive in HTLV EIA and confirmed as positive in more specific testing should be permanently deferred.[56] These individuals should be informed of their test results and receive counseling for the meaning of a positive test result. If a person's serum specimen is repeatably reactive in EIA, the person should not be notified of the test result unless the test result is repeatably reactive on two separate donations. When this occurs the person should be informed of the test result and discouraged from donating blood. However, the donors should not be informed that they are infected with HTLV-I or HTLV-II, because the meaning of this type of test result is not known.[56] Persons seropositive for HTLV-I should be counseled as to the meaning of the test result and the disease risks of HTLV-I infection. In the process of counseling, every effort should be made to stress the following points: (i) the current estimated risk of disease (either ATLL or HAM/TSP) in an HTLV-I-infected population is approximately 1% to 4% (96–99% of infected individuals remain asymptomatic throughout their lifetime); (ii) that HTLV-I is a retrovirus, but not the AIDS virus, and that the test result does not imply the person has AIDS; (iii) blood, plasma, organ, or sperm donations should not be made; (iv) the person should not share needles or syringes or other paraphernalia of any kind after parenteral injections; (v) breast-feeding of infants should not be performed; and (vi) a physician should be consulted concerning appropriate precautions to prevent sexual transmission of the virus to another person. To reduce the probability of sexual transmission of the virus, an infected person should not engage in sexual intercourse with multiple

TABLE 12.7. Recommendations for persons seropositive for HTLV-I[a].

1. Consult physician concerning HTLV-I disease associations, etc. Counseling physician should minimize anxiety and clearly indicate risk of development of HTLV-I-related diseases (e.g., 1–4% of infected individuals over their lifetime ever develop disease, and HTLV-II infection has not been clearly linked with human disease).
2. Do not donate blood, plasma, organs, tissue, or sperm.
3. Do not share needles, syringes, or other instruments used for injections.
4. Females should not breast-feed infants.
5. Sexual transmission has been documented for HTLV-I, and a health care person provided should be consulted about precautions to prevent sexual transmission of HTLV-I to another person.

[a] Adapted from Kaplan J, Khabbaz R. HTLV-I: Newest addition to blood donor screening. Am Fam physician 1989;40:189–195.

partners, and males should use a condom to reduce the risk of transmission of the infection (Table 12.7).[56]

References

1. Poiesz B, Ruscetti F, Gazdar A, Bunn P, Mina J, Gallo R. Detection and isolation of type C retrovirus particles from fresh and cultured lymphocytes of patients with cutaneous T-cell lymphoma. Proc Natl Acad Sci USA 1980;77: 7415–7419.
2. Gessain A, Barin F, Vernant J, Gout O, Maurs L, Calender A, de The G. Antibodies to human T lymphotropic virus type 1 in patients with tropical spastic paresis. Lancet 1985;ii:407–410.
3. Osame M, Usuku K, Izumo S, Ijichi N, Amitani H, Igata A, Matusumoto M, Tara M. HTLV-I associated myelopathy: a new clinical entity. Lancet 1986; i:1031–1032.
4. Morgan O, Mora C, Rodgers-Johnson P, Char G. HTLV-I and polymyositis in Jamaica. Lancet 1989;8673:1184–1186.
5. Nishioka K, Maruyama I, Sato K, Kitajima I, Nkajima Y, Osame M. Chronic inflammatory anrthropathy associated with HTLV-I. Lancet 1989;8635: 441.
6. Kalyanaraman V, Sarngadharan M, Robert-Guroff M, Miyoshi I, Golde D, Gallo R. A new subtype of human T-cell leukemia virus (HTLV-II) associated with a T-cell variant of hairy cell leukemia. Science 1982;218:571–573.
7. Lairmore M, Jacobson S, Gracia F, De B, Castillo L, Larreategui M, Roberts B, Levine P, Blattner W, Kaplan J. Isolation of human T-lymphotropic virus type 2 from Guaymi indians in Panama. Proc Natl Acad Sci USA 1990;87: 8840–8844.
8. Lee H, Swanson P, Shorty V, Zack J, Rosenblatt J, Chen I. High rate of HTLV-II infection in seropositive IV drug abusers in New Orleans. Science 1989;244:471–475.

9. Papsidero L, Swartzwelder F, Sheu M, Montagna R, Ehrlich G, Bhagavati S, Dosik H, Sninsky J, Poiesz B. Immunodetection of human T-cell lymphotropic virus type 1 core protein in biological samples by using a monoclonal antibody immunoassay. J Clin Microbiol 1990;28:949–955.
10. De B, Srinivasan A. Multiple primer pairs for the detection of HTLV-I by PCR. Nucleic Acids Res 1989;17:2142.
11. Varmus H. Regulation of HIV and HTLV gene expression. Genes Dev 1988;2:1055–1062.
12. Green P, Chen I. Regulation of human T cell leukemia virus expression. FASEB J 1990;4:169–175.
13. Green J, Glenn B, Wagner D, Waldmann T, Jay G. Trans activation of granulocyte-macrophage colony stimulating factor and the interleukin-2 receptor in transgenic mice carrying the human T-lymphotropic virus type 1 tax gene. Mol Cell Biol 1989;9:4731–4737.
14. Fujii M, Sassone-Corsi P, Verma I. c-*fos* promoter transactivation by the tax1 protein of human T-cell leukemia virus type 1. Proc Natl Acad Sci USA 1988;85:8526–8530.
15. Leung K, Nabel G. HTLV-I transactivator induces expression through an NF-kappa B like factor. Nature (London) 1988;333:776–778.
16. Nerenbery M, Hinrichs S, Reynolds R, Khoury G, Jay G. The *tat* gene of human T-lymphotropic virus type 1 induces mesenchymal tumors in transgenic mice. Science 1987;237:1324–1329.
17. Kinoshita T, Shimoyama M, Tobinai K, Ito M, Shin-ichiro I, Ikeda S, Tajima K, Shimotohno K, Sugimua T. Detection of mRNA for the tax/rex gene of human T-cell leukemia virus type 1 in fresh peripheral blood mononuclear cells of adult T-cell leukemia patients and viral carriers by using the polymerase chain reaction. Proc Natl Acad Sci USA 1989;86:5620–5624.
18. Grassmann R, Dengler C, Muller-Fleckenstein I, Fleckenstein B, McGuire K, Dokhelar M-C, Sodroski J, Haseltine W. Transformation to continuous growth of primary human T lymphocytes by human T-cell leukemia virus type I X-region genes transduced by a herpesvirus saimiri vector. Proc Natl Acad Sci USA 1989;86:3351–3355.
19. Poteat H, Kadison P, McGuire K, Park L, Park R, Sodroski J, Haseltine W. Response of the human T-cell leukemia virus type 1 long terminal repeat to cyclic AMP. J Virol 1989;63:1604–1611.
20. Dodon M, Bernard A, Gazzolo L. Peripheral T-lymphocyte activation by human T-cell leukemia virus type 1 interferes with the CD2 but not with the CD3/TCR pathway. J Virol 1989;63:5413–5419.
21. Akizuki S, Setoguchi M, Nakazato O, Yoshida S, Higuchi Y, Yamamoto S, Okajima T. An autopsy case of human T-lymphotropic virus type 1-associated myelopathy. Hum Pathol 1988;19:988–990.
22. Moore W, Traugott U, Scheinberg L, Raine C. Tropical spastice paraparesis: a model of virus-induced, cytotoxic T-cell-mediated demyelination. Ann Neurol 1989;26:523–530.
23. Sawada M, Suzumura A, Yosida M, Marunouchi T. Human T-cell leukemia virus type 1 trans activator induces class I major histocompatibility complex antigen expression in glial cells. J Virol 1990;64:4002–4006.
24. Kuefler P, Bunn P. Adult T cell leukemia/lymphoma. Clin Haematol 1986; 15:695–708.

25. Richardson JH, Edwards AJ, Cruickshank JK, Rudge P, Dalgleish AG. In vivo cellular tropism of human T-cell leukemia virus type 1. J Virol 1990; 64:5682–5687.
26. Jacobson S, Raine CS, Mingioli ES, McFarlin DE. Isolation of an HTLV-1-like retrovirus from patients with tropical spastic paraparesis. Nature (London) 1988;331:540–543.
27. Daenke S, Nightingale S, Cruickshank J, Bangham C. Sequence variants of human T-cell lymphotropic virus type I from patients with tropical spastic paraparesis and adult T-cell leukemia do not distinguish neurological from leukemic isolates. J Virol 1990;64:1278–1282.
28. Blattner W. Retroviruses. In: Evans AS, ed. Viral Infections of Humans: Epidemiology and Control, 3d Ed. New York: Plenum, 1989:545–592.
29. Kajiyama W, Kashiwagi S, Ikematsu H, Jayahi J, Nomura H, Okochi K. Intrafamilial transmission of adult T cell leukemia virus. J Infect Dis 1986; 154:851–857.
30. Iwahara Y, Takehara N, Kataoka R, Sawada T, Ohtsuki Y, Nakachi H, Maehama T, Okayama T, Miyoshi I. Transmission of HTLV-I to rabbits via semen and breast milk from seropositive healthy persons. Int J Cancer 1990;45:980–983.
31. Miyoshi I, Fujishita M, Taguchi H, Matsubayashi K, Miwa N, Tanioka Y. Natural infection in nonhuman primates with adult T-cell leukemia virus or a closely related agent. Int J Cancer 1983;32:333–336.
32. Kinoshita K, Yamanouchi K, Ikeda S, Momita S, Amagasaki T, Soda H, Ichimaru M, Moriuchi R, Katamine S, Miyamoto T, Hino S. Oral infection of a common marmoset with human T-cell leukemia virus type 1 (HTLV-I) by inoculating fresh human milk of an HTLV-I carrier mother. Jpn J Cancer Res 1985;76:1147–1153.
33. Sugiyma H, Doi H, yamaguchi K, Tsuji Y, Miyamoto T, Hina S. Significance of postnatal mother to child transmission of human T-lymphotropic virus type 1 on the development of adult T-cell leukemia/lymphoma. J Med Virol 1986;20:253–258.
34. Saxton E, Lee H, Swanson P, Chen IS, Ruland C, Chin E, Aboulafia D, Delamarter R, Rosenblatt J. Detection of human T-cell leukemia/lymphoma virus type I in a transfusion recipient with chronic myelopathy. Neurology 1989;39:841–844.
35. Gout O, Baulac M, Gessain A, Semah F, Saal F, Peries J, Cabrol C, Foucault-Fretz C, Laplane D, Sigaux F, De The G. Rapid development of myelopathy after HTLV-I infection acquired by transfusion during cardiac transplantation. N Engl J Med 1990;322:383–388.
36. Centers for Disease Control. Licensure of screening tests for antibody to human T-lymphotropic virus type 1. MMWR 1988;37(48):736–747.
37. Williams A, Fang C, Salmon D, Poiesz B, Sandler G, Darr W, Shulman G, McGowan E, Douglas D, Bowman R, Peetoom F, Kleinman S, Lenes B, Dodd R. Seroprevalence and epidemiological correlates of HTLV-I infection in U.S. blood donors. Science 1988;240:643–646.
38. Lairmore M, Jason J, Hartley T, De B, Khabbaz, Evatt B. Absence of HTLV-I coinfection in HIV-infected hemophilic men. Blood 1989;74: 2596–2599.

39. Khabbaz R, Darrow W, Hartley T, Witte J, Cohen J, French J, Gill P, Potterat J, Sikes K, Reich R, Kaplan J, Lairmore M. Seroprevalence and risk factors for HTLV-I/II infection among female prosititutes in the United States. JAMA 1990;263:60–64.
40. Kelen GD, DiGiovanna TA, Lofy L, Junkin E, Stein A, Sivertson KT, Lairmore MD, Quinn TC. Human T-lymphotropic virus (HTLV 1/II) infection among patients in an inner-city emergency department. Ann Intern Med 1990;113:368–372.
41. Tschachler E, Robert-Guroff M, Gallo R, Reitz M. Human T-lymphotropic virus type I-infected T cells constitutively express lymphotoxin in vitro. Blood 1989;73:194–201.
42. Gessain A, Caudie C, Gout O, Vernant J, Maurs L, Giodan C, Tournier-Lasserve E, Essex M, de The G. Intrathecal synthesis of antibodies to human T lymphotropic virus type 1 and the presence of IgG oligoclonal bands in the cerebrospinal fluid of patients with endemic tropical spastic paraparesis. J Infect Dis 1988;157:1226–1234.
43. Itoyama Y, Minato S, Kira J, Goto I, Sato H, Okochi K, Yamamoto N. Spontaneous proliferation of peripheral blood lymphocytes increased in patients with HTLV-I-associated myelopathy. Neurology 1988;38:1302–1307.
44. Anderson DW, Epstein JS, Lee TH, Lairmore MD, Saxinger C, Kalyanaraman VS, Slamon D, Parks W, Poiesz BJ, Pierik LT, Lee H, Montagna R, Roche PA, Williams A, Blattner W. Serological confirmation of human T-lymphotropic virus type 1 infection in healthy blood and plasma donors. Blood 1989;74:2585–2591.
45. Hartley T, Khabbaz R, Cannon R, Kaplan J, Lairmore M. Characterization of antibody reactivity to human T-cell lymphotropic virus types 1 and 2 using immunoblot and radioimmunoprecipitation assays. J Clin Microbiol 1990;28: 646–650.
46. Palker T, Scearce E, Ho W, Copeland T, Oroszlan S, Popovic N, Haynes B. Monoclonal antibodies reactive with human T cell lymphotropic virus I (HTLV-I) p19 internal core protein: cross reactivity with normal tissues and differential reactivity with HTLV types I and II. J Immunol 1985;135:247–254.
47. Gallo D, Diggs JL, Hanson CV. Comparison of western immunoblot antigens and interpretive criteria for detection of antibody to human T-lymphotropic virus types I and II. J Clin Microbiol 1990;28:2045–2050.
48. Khabbaz RF, Hartley TM, Lairmore MD, Kaplan JE. Epidemiologic assessment of screening tests for antibody to human T-lymphotropic virus type 1 (HTLV-I). Am J Public Health 1990;80:190–192.
49. Coates SR, Harris AJ, Parkes DL, Smith CM, Liu H-L, Akita RW, Ferrer MM, Sampson EK, Brandis JW, Sliwkowski MX. Serological evaluation of *Escherichia coli*-expressed human T-cell leukemia virus type 1 env, gag p24, and tax proteins. J Clin Microbiol 1990;28:1139–1142.
50. Chen Y-M, Lee T-H, Samuel KP, Okayama A, Tachibana N, Miyoshi I, Papas TS, Essex M. Antibody reactivity to different regions of human T-cell leukemia type 1 gp61 in infected people. J Virol 1989;63:4952–4957.
51. Thorn RM, Braman WM, Beltz GA, Wilde A, Hung C-H, Seals J, Marciani D. Initial evaluation of a recombinant HTLV-I gp21 enzyme immunoassay.

In: Blattner W, ed. *Human Retrovirology: HTLV*. New York: Raven, 1990: 419–422.

52. Lal R, Rudolph D, Lairmore M, Khabbaz R, Garfield M, Coligan J, Folks T. Serologic discrimination of HTLV-I and HTLV-II infection by using a synthetic peptide based enzyme immunoassay. J Infect Dis 1991;163:41–46.
53. Lipka JJ, Bui K, Reyes GR, Moeckli R, Wiktor SZ, Blattner WA, Murphy EL, Shaw GM, Hanson CV, Sninsky JJ, Foung S. Determination of a unique and immunodominant epitope of human T-cell lymphotropic virus type 1. J Infect Dis 1990; 162:353–357.
54. Kaplan M, Marselle LM, Pahwa SG, Chayt KJ, Sarngadharan MG, Wong-Staal, Gallo R. Concomitant infection with HTLV-I and HTLV-III in a patient with T8 lymphoproliferative disease. N Engl J Med 1986;315:1073–1078.
55. Yamaguchi K, Seiki M, Yoshida M, Nishimura H, Kawano F, Takatsuki K. The detection of human T cell leukemia virus proviral DNA and its application for classification and diagnosis of T cell malignancy. Blood 1984;63:1235–1240.
56. Kaplan JE, Khabbaz RF. HTLV-I: newest addition to blood donor screening. Am Fam Physician 1989;40:189–195.

13
Biosafety: Principles and Practices in the Human Immunodeficiency Virus Laboratory

M. E. KENNEDY

Safe methods for the containment and handling of potentially infectious materials is a widely recognized need in the management of diagnostic, clinical and research laboratories. Such management is often focused on laboratories primarily involved in the manipulation of infectious agents for the purpose of diagnosis or research. In other areas of the health care system where blood, tissue, secreta, or excreta are analyzed, such as biochemistry, hematology or toxicology laboratories, safety management is often a low priority. In such laboratories, specific training and education of the technician is often in the field of molecular biology or immunology, with little or no background in the pathogenic microbiology. The hazards of handling infectious material are often unrecognized and poorly understood. Basic protective measures and equipment when appropriately applied, however, will provide a safe working environment in all types of laboratories.

Laboratory-Acquired Infections

Infections among laboratorians have a long and varied history. As early as 1893 the literature reports laboratory-acquired typhoid fever[1]; fungal infections were reported in 1903[2]; typhus in 1910[3]; and the first recorded laboratory-acquired hepatitis in 1929.[4] Subsequent studies including that of Lauer et al.,[5] firmly established that laboratory infections with hepatitis resulted from contact with infected material or by ingestion or injection. Other agents are found in human blood and have been associated with blood transfusions. These include human immunodeficiency virus (HIV), cylomegalovirus, Epstein–Barr virus, pseudomonas, syphilis, relapsing fever, leptospirosis, and protozoan infections including malaria, babesiasis, toxoplasmosis, trypanosomiasis, leishmaniasis, and filariasis, Rocky Mountain spotted fever and Q fever.[6]

Although these agents have caused infection by a restricted mode of transmission (transfusion), it is not unreasonable to assume that they could also be transmitted to a laboratory worker by accidental parenteral injection of blood, by contamination of cuts or abrasions, or by ingestion. Hence, the spectrum of agents to which the laboratorian is exposed is indeed large, as are other factors that expose the laboratory worker to biohazardous agents found in blood. A study by Evans et al.[7] assayed 800 environmental samples from 10 clinical or research laboratories and found that 31 samples contained hepatitis B virus surface antigen (HBgAg). High workloads, inappropriate behavior, and flawed laboratory techniques were identified as contributing factors.

The route of exposure, the infectious dose, and the susceptibility of the host all play a significant role in the initiation of infection. Particular concern has been expressed most often by laboratory and other health care workers of the possibility of contracting acquired immunodeficiency syndrome (AIDS) or hepatitis (HBV). HBV as an occupationally acquired disease may be present in blood in concentrations up to 10^9 viral particles per milliliter[8] whereas HIV is usually found in concentrations of 10–50 viral particles per milliliter of serum from infectious patients.[9] In addition to blood, HIV has been isolated from semen, vaginal secretions, saliva, tears, breast milk, cerebrospinal fluid, amniotic fluid, alveolar fluid, and urine; thus, exposure or transmission is possible from any of these specimens in a clinical or laboratory setting.

Current information indicates that the infection rate of HIV in laboratory workers is low. The consequences of infection however are dire and must not be underestimated. Canadian statistics provided by the Federal Centre for AIDS from September 1985 to May 1990 have recorded to date 336 exposures to HIV-infected blood or body fluids (Table 13.1). To date, there have been no Canadian seroconversions among employees enrolled in this program. Data from the World Health Organization[9] show transmission of HIV can and does occur in health care settings. Table 13.2 lists the type of procedure and the potential of risk of HIV exposure to laboratory and health care personnel. Table 13.3 lists cases for whom seroconversion was documented after a specific exposure. Safe work practices and appropriate protective equipment remain, today, the only protection available against job-related HIV infection. These together with constant vigilance and training in safe practices become paramount in providing a safe working environment and reducing the potential exposure to HIV and other infectious agents in the health care setting.

Basic Safety Measures

The following requirements are basic to the safe operation of a laboratory handling infectious or potentially infectious materials including those previously discussed.

TABLE 13.1. Exposures by occupation group (September 1985–May 1990)[a].

	Nurse	Laboratory technician	Other	Therapist/ technician	Student/ resident	Physician	Total
Needle-stick	127	14	8	6	13	9	177 (53%)
Scalpel wound	11	3	2	0	1	1	18 (5%)
Eye-splash	24	4	1	6	1	2	38 (11%)
Open wound contamination	30	5	3	2	1	1	42 (13%)
Skin contact:							
Intact	2	1	3	1	0	1	8 (2%)
Nonintact	6	4	1	1	0	1	13 (4%)
Unknown	33	2	3	2	0	0	40 (12%)
	233 (69%)	33 (10%)	21 (6%)	18 (5%)	16 (5%)	15 (4%)	336 (100%)

[a] Source: Federal Centre for AIDS, Health and Welfare Canada.

TABLE 13.2. Potential HIV exposure.[a]

Procedure	Person at risk	Mode of transmission
Blood sample collection	Patient	Contaminated needle Contaminated hands or gloves of phlebotomist Skin puncture by needle or broken container
Specimen transfer	Laboratory personnel Transport worker	Broken or contaminated exterior of container Spill or splash of specimen
Specimen manipulation	Laboratory personnel	Skin puncture contamination Contaminated or broken specimen container Contaminated work surface Specimen spills or splashes Perforated gloves
Cleaning and maintenance	Laboratory personnel Support staff	Skin puncture or contamination Splashes or spills Contaminated work surfaces
Waste disposal	Laboratory personnel Support staff Transport worker Public	Puncture wounds and cuts Skin contamination

[a] Adapted from Centers for Disease Control and National Institutes of Health.[12]

Eating, smoking, drinking, or applying cosmetics must not be permitted in the laboratory. Food items should be stored in designated refrigerators, away from the work area.

Laboratory coats, gowns, etc. should be worn when working with the infectious or potentially infectious materials and removed when leaving the work area. Laboratory clothing must not be worn in cafeterias, lunch or smoking rooms, toilets, etc.

Laboratory staff must wash their hands after handling infectious or potentially infectious materials or animals and bedding and before leaving the laboratory.

Mouth-pipetting of any liquid in the laboratory must not be permitted. Mechanical pipetting devices must be used.

Care should be taken to avoid skin contact with infectious materials or articles exposed to them. Disposable gloves are recommended.

Extraordinary care must be taken to avoid wounds from sharp instruments. Disposable needles and syringes are preferred. Only needle-locking syringes should be used. Needles should not be bent, sheared, or replaced into their sheath. Needles and syringes should be disposed of in puncture-proof containers by autoclaving or incineration.

TABLE 13.3. Worldwide HIV seroconversions in health care workers.[a]

Date	Country	Type of exposure	Number
1984	United Kingdom	Needle-stick	1
1986	United States	Cutaneous	1
		Needle-stick	1
	Martinique	Needle-stick	1
	France	Needle-stick	1
1987	United States	Needle-stick	1
		Nonintact skin	2
		Mucous membrane	1
1988	United States	Needle-stick(s)	5
		Sharp object(s)	2
	France	Needle-stick	1
	Italy	Mucous membrane	1

[a] Adapted from WHO Bull 1989;67(5):577–582.

Necropsy of laboratory animals should be performed whenever possible in biological safety cabinets. Full protective laboratory clothing including full face protection and double gloves should be worn.

Laboratory procedures should be performed to minimize the production of aerosols. Certified biological safety cabinets (Class I or II) or other containment devices should be used as primary containment for *all* procedures with a potential for the creation of aerosols. These include centrifuging, blending, mixing, sonicating, and harvesting infected tissue or cultures.

All work surfaces must be decontaminated daily or when knowingly contaminated, using an effective surface disinfectant. (Widely recommended is a 1:10 dilution of household bleach containing approximately 5.25% sodium hypochlorite.)

All contaminated or potentially contaminated wastes from the laboratories and animal rooms must be decontaminated, preferably by autoclaving or incineration, before disposal.

All laboratory spills, accidents, or overt or potential exposures to infectious materials must be reported immediately. Appropriate medical evaluation and treatment must be available and provided to staff.

Baseline serum samples from laboratory employees should be collected and stored, initially on employment and then periodically thereafter.

Biosafety Requirements for HIV Serology Laboratories

In addition to the requirements listed under basic safety measures, the following are appropriate for working with specimens requiring serological procedures.

The laboratory room(s) should be away from public areas, offices, or patient care areas. If possible, a dedicated room should be provided to perform serological procedures on specimens potentially infectious with HIV.

Protective laboratory clothing, such as disposable gowns, rubber or latex gloves, and safety glasses should be provided.

Biological safety cabinets are not required for serological testing procedures unless they create aerosols. For procedures in which splashes may occur, protective barriers, such as plastic countertop shields, should be provided.

Full face shields or other protective devices should be worn to protect the operator against activities that may create splashes of blood or other contaminated fluids, such as opening vacuum blood tubes.

Standard laboratory furnishings that are readily cleanable and capable of disinfection should be used.

Foot- and hand-operated handwashing sinks, preferably dedicated to this purpose, should be located at the exit to the serology laboratory.

Specialized room ventilation is not required. If windows that are openable are provided, they must be provided with screening.

All laboratory room doors must be self-closing and remain closed during working hours.

An autoclave for decontamination of laboratory wastes should be in or near the laboratory working area. If materials are disposed of by incineration, they must be removed from the laboratory in sealed leakproof containers.

Biosafety Requirements for HIV Isolation Laboratories

The operational requirements in this type of laboratory are substantially more stringent than previously described. The laboratory staff must receive specific training in the safe handling and manipulation of viral agents that are isolated. The following requirements apply.

The isolation laboratory must be an area dedicated for work with HIV-contaminated material. Access to this laboratory should be restricted to necessary personnel *only*.

Dedicated solid-front laboratory clothing is worn in the virus isolation laboratory and is removed before leaving the laboratory. Laboratory clothing is autoclaved before laundering.

Procedures for isolation, including manipulating infected cell cultures and concentrated viral preparations, must be performed in a certified biological safety cabinet.

Centrifugation is carried out in sealed buckets or heads that are loaded and unloaded in the biological safety cabinet.

A foot, knee, or automatically operated handwashing sink should be provided at the exit of the laboratory.

Biosafety Requirements for HIV Research and Production Laboratories

Research and production laboratories require personnel who are highly skilled and well versed in both the procedures of the laboratory operation and the equipment used therein. Access to this area is physically restricted, and protocols for work practices, accidents, and emergencies are thoroughly defined. The requirements of these laboratories are strengthened because of manipulation or production of concentrated viral preparations. In addition to the biosafety requirements or serological or viral isolation laboratories, the following are required.

Entrance to the laboratory area must be restricted by requiring passage through two sets of doors which are lockable.

Windows of the laboratory must be closed and sealed.

All penetrations to the room perimeter, including those in the walls, ceiling, and floor, are sealed.

A sealed, ducted mechanical ventilation system must be provided that ensures directional (inward) airflows at all times. High-efficiency particulate airfilters (HEPA) may or may not be required. The air supply system must be interlocked with the exhaust system to prevent pressurization of the laboratory in the event of exhaust fan failure.

An autoclave must be located in or adjacent to the research or production facility.

It is recommended that all staff be offered a yearly medical examination and provide serum, samples for storage.

It is highly recommended that all staff be offered the hepatitis B vaccine.

The combination of physical containment with good laboratory practices will minimize the potential for exposure to HIV and other infectious agents in the workplace. Readers are encouraged to refer to published biosafety guidelines[10–14] for specific details on containment equipment, facility design, medical surveillance, waste management, disinfection, and sterilization. The constant training of staff and strict adherence to good laboratory practices remain paramount in achieving a safe working environment in the microbiology laboratory.

References

1. Kisskalt K. Laboratoriumsinfektionen mit Typhusbazillen. Z Hyg Infektionskr 1915;50:145–162.
2. Evan N. A clinical report of a case of blastomycosis of the skin from accidental inoculation. JAMA 1903;40:1772–1775.

3. Collins CH. Laboratory-Acquired Infections. 2d Ed. London: Butterworth, 1988.
4. Donovan JW. The first case of laboratory acquired hepatitis? Trans R Soc Trop Med Hyg 1974;68:259.
5. Lauer JL, Van Drunen NA, Washburn JW, Balfour HH. Transmission of hepatitis B virus in clinical laboratory areas. J Infect Dis 1979;140:513–576.
6. Sandler SG, Schorr JB. Acquired immunodeficiency syndrome and other transfusion-transmissible diseases. In Kasprisin L., ed. Pediatric Transfusion Medicine, Vol. II. Florida: CRC Press, 1988.
7. Evans MR, Henderson DK, Bennett JE. Potential for laboratory exposures to biohazardous agents found in blood. Am J Public Health 1990;80:423–427.
8. Almeida JD. Individual morphological variations seen in Australian antigen positive sera. Am J Dis Child 1972;123:303–309.
9. Levy JA. Human immunodeficiency viruses and the pathogenisis of AIDS. JAMA 1989;261:2997–3006.
10. Marcus R, Kay K, Mann JM. Transmission of human immunodeficiency virus (HIV) in health-care settings worldwide. Bull WHO 1989;67(5):577–582.
11. Medical Research Council of Canada/Laboratory Centre for Disease Control, Health and Welfare Canada. Laboratory Biosafety guidelines. Canada: Minister of Supply and Services Canada, 1990.
12. Centers for Disease Control and National Institutes of Health. Biosafety in Microbiological and Biomedical Laboratories. 2d Ed. Washington, DC: U.S. Dept. of Health and Human Services, 1988.
13. Biosafety Guidelines for Diagnostic and Research Laboratories Working with HIV. Global Programme on AIDS. Geneva: World Health Organization, in press.
14. HIV—The Causative Agent of AIDS and Related Conditions. 2nd rev. Merseyside: Health and Safety Executive, 1990.

14 Management of Occupational Exposure to the Human Immunodeficiency Virus

KENNETH G. CASTRO and JACQUELYN A. POLDER

Much concern exists among health care workers about the possibility of occupational acquisition of human immunodeficiency virus (HIV) infection. Throughout the United States, several hundred health care workers who have experienced documented exposures to blood or other body fluids of persons infected with HIV have been followed prospectively. Results from these studies have demonstrated that the risk of HIV transmission associated with a single percutaneous exposure is on the average 0.33% (approximately 1 infection for every 350 exposures).[1–4] Most efforts to prevent occupational HIV infection have focused on universal infection control precautions to reduce the incidence of occupational exposures.[5] Strict adherence to these recommendations will reduce, but may not completely eliminate, the risk of such exposures. Additional recommendations have been made for management of health care workers following occupational exposure to blood from HIV-infected patients.[6,7] This chapter focuses on elements of postexposure management and discusses issues regarding the use of prophylactic zidovudine.

General Principles

Employers should make available to health care workers a system for prompt evaluation following an occupational exposure to HIV. Worker education is an integral component of such a system (Table 14.1), and it should be included in the workers' orientation and ongoing inservice educational activities. One of the goals of such programs is to familiarize workers with their personal risk of occupational exposure to HIV. To provide clear guidance and avoid undue concern, each institution should adopt a definition of what constitutes an occupational exposure that may place a worker at risk of HIV infection.

The U.S. Public Health Service has defined such an exposure as

> "a percutaneous injury (e.g., a needlestick or cut with a sharp object), contact of mucous membranes, or contact of skin (especially when the exposed skin is

TABLE 14.1. List of objectives in educational program for health-care workers.

I. Prevention Component
   A. Describe blood and body fluids requiring universal precautions.
   B. Describe and be familiar with universal precautions.
   C. Know where to access materials necessary for universal precautions (e.g., gloves, gowns, puncture-proof containers)
   D. Follow universal precautions routinely.

II. Management Component
   A. Define occupational exposure.
   B. Become familiar with personal risk of occupational exposure and preventive actions.
   F. Become familiar with postexposure management program and steps to be followed on occurrence of incident (include ready access to emergency telepone numbers).
   G. Discuss postexposure management options, including theoretic basis of postexposure zidovudine prophylaxis, its availability, side effects, and need for follow-up.

chapped, abraded, or afflicted with dermatitis or the contact is prolonged or involving an extensive area) with blood, tissues, or other body fluids to which universal precautions apply, including: a) semen, vaginal secretions, or other body fluids contaminated with visible blood, because these substances have been implicated in the transmission of HIV infection; b) cerebrospinal fluid, synovial fluid, pleural fluid, peritoneal fluid, pericardial fluid, and amniotic fluid, because the risk of HIV transmission from these fluids has not yet been determined; and c) laboratory specimens that contain HIV (e.g., suspensions of concentrated virus)."[6]

The worksite orientation and educational activities should include opportunities to openly discuss the risks and actions to be undertaken in the event of an occupational exposure. Employees must be trained to report exposures immediately after they occur, because certain interventions that may be appropriate must be initiated promptly to be effective. Most consultants agree that the postexposure period is not the optimal time to first consider the use of zidovudine.

After an occupational exposure, exposed employees and source individuals should be evaluated to determine the possible need for prophylaxis against hepatitis B virus (HBV) infection and the need for follow-up serologic testing for HIV antibody (e.g., baseline, 6, 12, and 24 weeks after exposure). If consent cannot be obtained from the source individual, policies should be developed for testing source individuals in compliance with applicable state and local laws. Confidentiality of the exposed worker and the source individual must be safeguarded at all times. Existing guidelines recommend that if an exposure occurs, the circumstances should be recorded in a confidential medical record. Relevant information includes: date and time of exposure; job duty being performed at time of exposure; details of exposure (amount and type of fluid or material, severity of exposure); description of source of exposure (and HIV or HBV status, if known); and details about counseling, post-exposure management, and follow-up plans.[6] This system of evaluation and follow-up should be available at all times when employees may be exposed to blood or body fluids.

Emergency Treatment

Each incident of occupational exposure to blood or body fluids requiring universal precautions should be treated by employees as a medical emergency. After an occupational exposure, first aid should be administered as necessary (including wound cleansing and irrigation with soap and water), and both the exposed worker and the source individual should be evaluated to determine the possible need for the exposed worker to receive prophylaxis against HBV infection. Ideally, all health care workers should be immunized against HBV. If the HIV or HBV antibody status of the source individual is unknown, informed consent should be obtained and blood drawn for both HIV and HBV antibody testing. Appropriate medical referral, counseling, and advice regarding risk of occupational transmission of either HIV or HBV should be promptly available (e.g., available within an hour of exposure). This is likely to require the implementation of an on-call system.

Considerations Regarding Zidovudine Prophylaxis

Zidovudine (azidothymidine, AZT) is a thymidine analogue that has been shown in vitro to inhibit replication of HIV by interfering with the action of viral RNA-dependent DNA polymerase (reverse transcriptase).[8] Zidovudine has been shown to increase the length and quality of life of patients with advanced AIDS-related complex (ARC) and AIDS.[9] Additionally, zidovudine has been shown to retard progression to advanced AIDS in ARC patients and asymptomatic individuals with CD4 lymphocyte counts under 500/mm^3.[10,11] The efficacy of zidovudine prophylaxis for humans after exposure to HIV cannot be ascertained, however, because of insufficient data.

Some institutions have offered zidovudine as prophylaxis against HIV infection to persons after certain occupational exposures to blood or body fluids known to be infected with HIV. The theoretical rationale for post-exposure zidovudine use are based on the antiviral effect of zidovudine in the treatment of persons with established HIV infection, the apparent reversibility of acute toxicity in persons taking zidovudine for a brief period, and the suggestion that in studies using mice and cats, administration of zidovudine shortly after exposure to other animal retroviruses appeared to modify or prevent retroviral infection.[12–14] Additionally, suppression of HIV infection has been demonstrated in SCID-hu mice following postexposure administration of 250 mg/kg/day of zidovudine within 2 hours of infection.[15] However, limited studies involving primates have not shown success with zidovudine in postexposure prophylaxis against simian immunodeficiency virus (SIV).[16] Three brief reports have documented the failure of postexposure zidovudine in preventing HIV infection in three persons who experienced percutaneous exposure to blood contaminated with HIV.[17,18,19]

In the first case report, an HIV-uninfected patient accidentally received by intravenous injection approximately 100–200 μl of blood from a man infected with HIV-1. Zidovudine was begun 45 minutes post exposure at a dose of 500 mg orally every 6 hours and continued for 2 days, followed by 2.5 mg per kilogram of body weight intravenously from day 3 to day 20, and then 500 mg orally every 6 hours from day 21 to day 37. The patient continued to receive 250 mg of zidovudine orally every 6 hours for the next two months. HIV-1 p24 antigen was detected in blood samples obtained from the exposed patient on the 30th day post exposure, and HIV-1 antibody was present on day 41.[17]

In the second case report, a heath care worker sustained "a deep needlestick injury after taking blood from a patient with AIDS." Zidovudine was started within 6 hours of the accident at a dose of 250 mg orally every 6 hours and continued for 8 weeks. Blood obtained from the health care worker shortly after the exposure was negative for antibody to HIV-1. Five weeks later, the worker experienced an influenza-like illness, and on the sixth week HIV-1 antibody was detected.[18]

The third report was a suicide attempt by a woman who inoculated herself (exact route not specified) with 2 to 3 ml of blood from a former male friend with AIDS. Two hours later she sought medical attention. Zidovudine prophylaxis was reportedly "immediately begun" with 250 mg orally every 6 hours and continued for 5 weeks. Blood samples obtained at baseline and four weeks after the incident were negative for HIV-1 and HIV-2 antibodies. Three months later she experienced lymphadenopathy, and was found to have antibody to HIV-1 ten days after the onset of this clinical syndrome.[19]

The Burroughs-Wellcome Company sponsored a study to evaluate the side effects and efficacy of postexposure zidovudine use. Preliminary results showed that some persons experienced mild reversible side effects when given 200 mg orally every 4 hours for 6 weeks (see side effects, following), and no instances of HIV-1 infection were detected.[20] However, because of the relative infrequency of HIV transmission after a single percutaneous exposure, the results regarding efficacy are inconclusive. Tokars and colleagues[1] estimated that more than 2,400 persons exposed to HIV would need to be followed prospectively to observe a statistically significant event if postexposure zidovudine is assumed to prevent 75% of occupational HIV transmission, given an estimated 0.33%

HIV transmission rate from such exposures. Evidently, if the chemoprophylactic outcome of zidovudine is less than 75% effective, a much larger cohort of exposed persons would need to be followed.

Although the efficacy of zidovudine prophylaxis in HIV exposures is ultimately not known, some expert consultants recommend that, if zidovudine is used for this purpose, it should be administered shortly after an exposure (within a few hours) because human HIV infection probably becomes established within hours of exposure. The U.S. Food and Drug Administration (FDA) has recognized that zidovudine effectively blocks the replication of HIV and has approved its use for certain patients with symptomatic and asymptomatic HIV infections. The FDA, however, has not approved zidovudine for marketing as a treatment to prevent infection following a documented occupational exposure. Therefore, individuals should recognize that such use would constitute the use of an approved drug for an unlabeled indication.

Because no definitive information is available on efficacy if zidovudine is used as prophylaxis, a dosage and duration of schedule must be established by the prescribing physician and the exposed worker. Different schedules are currently offered by various institutions. At the National Institutes of Health, employees who elect to receive zidovudine post exposure are given two 100 mg capsules by mouth every 4 hours (six times daily) for 42 days (6 weeks). At San Francisco General Hospital, employees who elect to receive zidovudine post exposure are given two 100 mg capsules by mouth every 4 hours (five times daily; no dose is given at 4:00 A.M.) for 28 days (4 weeks).[7] Regardless of the schedule selected, exposed individuals should receive appropriate medical follow-up care to monitor for drug toxicity.

Some of the well-recognized, short-term, reversible side effects of zidovudine therapy include headache, nausea, vomiting, diarrhea, hepatitis, insomnia, myalgia, anemia, and leukopenia. Long-term side effects are unknown, but could possibly include carcinogenic and teratogenic effects. Vaginal tumors, including carcinomas, have been observed in mice (and rats) receiving doses of zidovudine that the FDA has determined resulted in plasma levels in mice approximately equal to human plasma levels at the dose originally approved for treatment of persons with symptomatic HIV infection (200 mg every 4 hours).[6]

It is not known whether zidovudine can cause fetal harm when administered to pregnant women or whether it can affect reproductive capacity. For these reasons, it is recommended that women be evaluated for pregnancy before administration of zidovudine and that pregnancy be avoided throughout the time zidovudine is taken. Effective contraception can be achieved either by sexual abstinence or the use of latex condoms. It is also not known whether zidovudine is excreted in human milk. Because HIV can be transmitted through breast milk, exposed mothers should be informed of this risk and suggested to discontinue breast-

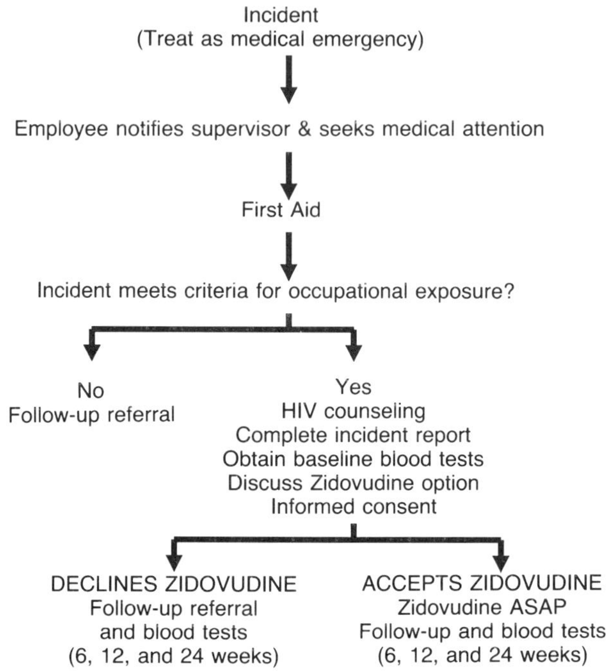

FIGURE 14.1. Guidelines for management of occupational exposures to HIV, including considerations for zidovudine use.

feeding whether or not they are receiving zidovudine. In the absence of definitive data on efficacy, safety, and toxicity, the decision to use zidovudine after exposure should ultimately rest with the exposed worker.

Following an exposure, the exposed worker should receive counseling regarding (i) the risk of occupational HIV infection; (ii) the theoretical rationale for postexposure zidovudine use; (iii) the side effects associated with drug use; (iv) advice to prevent further HIV transmission to a sexual partner or offspring in the event the employee became infected; (v) follow-up and drug dosage explanations; and (vi) plans to safeguard confidentiality of the employee and source individual. Signed informed consent should reflect the information covered during the counseling session. An outline of actions to be undertaken after an occupational exposure to HIV is shown in Figure 14.1. Workers at risk for such exposures need to be familiar with available mechanisms to promptly notify employers and to receive immediate attention, evaluation, and appropriate follow-up. In many instances, this implies having zidovudine available at the worksite by a designated physician or other health care provider.

Surveillance of Workers with Occupational Exposures to HIV

Additional data are needed to evaluate the efficacy of postexposure prophylaxis, establish the optimal dosage, define the optimal duration of prophylaxis, and define the duration of follow-up needed to detect HIV infection in persons who elect to receive prophylaxis. To collect additional information on postexposure chemoprophylaxis with zidovudine (or other antiretroviral agents), the Centers for Disease Control (CDC) has expanded its onging surveillance of workers with occupational exposures to HIV. No names or other personal identifiers are collected. All physicians who provide care to a worker within 1 month after an occupational exposure to HIV are encouraged to enroll the worker in the CDC surveillance system. Additional information and enrollment materials can be obtained from the Hospital Infections Program, Center for Infectious Diseases, Centers for Disease Control, Atlanta, Georgia 30333 (U.S.A.); telephone (404) 639-1547.

References

1. Tokars JI, Marcus RA, Culver DH, McKibben PS, Bell DM. Zidovudine (AZT) use after occupational exposure to HIV-infected blood. In Interscience Conference on Antimicrobial Agents and Chemotherapy, Atlanta, Georgia, 1990:168 (abstr. 490).
2. Marcus R, CDC Cooperative Needlestick Study Group. Surveillance of health-care workers exposed to blood from patients infected with the human immunodeficiency virus. N Engl J Med 1988;319:1118–1123.
3. Gerberding JL, Bryant-LeBlanc CE, Nelson K, Moss AR, Osmond D, Carlson JR, Drew ML, Levy JA, Sande MA. Risk of transmitting the human immunodeficiency virus, cytomegalovirus, and hepatitis B virus to health care workers exposed to patients with AIDS and AIDS-related conditions. J Infect Dis 1987;156:1–7.
4. Henderson DK. HIV-1 in the health care setting. In Mandell GF, Douglas RG, Jr, Bennett JE, eds. Principles and Practice of Infectious Diseases. 3rd Ed. New York: Churchill Livingstone, 1990:2221–2236.
5. CDC. Recommendations for prevention for HIV transmission in health-care settings. MMWR 1987;36(no.2S).
6. CDC. Public Health Service statement on management of occupational exposure to human immunodeficiency virus, including considerations regarding zidovudine postexposure use. MMWR 1990;39(RR-1).
7. Henderson DK, Gerberding JL. Prophylactic zidovudine after occupational exposure to the human immunodeficiency virus: an interim analysis. J Infect Dis 1989;160:321–327.
8. Yarchoan R, Mitsuya H, Myers C, Broder S. Clinical pharmacology of 3′-azido-2′, 3′-dideoxythimidine (zidovudine) and related dideoxynucleosides. N Engl J Med 1989;321:726–738.

9. Fischl MA, Richman DD, Grieco MH, Gottlieb MS, Volberding PA, Laskin OL, et al. The efficacy of azidothymidine (AZT) in the treatment of patients with AIDS and AIDS-related complex. N Engl J Med 1987;317:185–191.
10. Volberding PA, Lagakos SW, Koch MA, Pettinelli C, Myers MW, Booth DK, et al. Zidovudine in asymptomatic human immunodeficiency virus infection. N Engl J Med 1990;322:941–949.
11. Fischl MA, Richman DD, Hansen M, Collier AC, Carey JT, Para MF, et al. The safety and efficiency of zidovudine (AZT) in the treatment of subjects with mildly symptomatic human immunodeficiency virus type-1 (HIV) infection. Ann Intern Med 1990;112:727–737.
12. Ruprecht RM, O'Brien LG, Rossoni LD, Nusinoff-Lehrman S. Suppression of mouse viraemia and retroviral disease by 3′-azido-3′-deoxithymidine. Nature (London) 1986;323:467–469.
13. Tavares L, Roneker C, Johnston K, Nusinoff-Lehrman S, de Noronha F. 3′-Azido-3′-deoxithymidine in feline leukemia virus-infected cats: a model for therapy and prophylaxis of AIDS. Cancer Res 1987;47:3190–3194.
14. McCune JM, Namikawa R, Shih CC, Rabin LR, Kaneshima H. Suppression of HIV infection in AZT-treated SCID-hu mice. Science 1990;247:564–566.
15. Shih C-C, Kaneshima H, Rabin L, Namikawa R, Sager P, McGowan J, McCune JM. Postexposure prophylaxis with zidovudine suppresses human immunodeficiency virus type 1 infection in SCID-hu mice in a time-dependent manner. J Infect Dis 1991:163:625–627.
16. McClure HM, Anderson DC, Fultz P, Ansari A, Brodie A, Lehrman A. Prophylactic effects of AZT following exposure of macaques to an acutely lethal variant of SIV (SIV/SMM/PBj-14). In Abstract, Vth international Conference on AIDS, Montreal, 1989:522.
17. Lange JMA, Boucher CAB, Hollak CEM, Wiltink EHH, Reiss P, van Royen EA, Roos M, Danner SA, Goudsmit J. Failure of prophylactic zidovudine after accidental exposure to HIV-1. N Engl J Med 1990;322:1375–1377.
18. Looke DF, Grove DI. Failed prophylactic zidovudine after needlestick injury. Lancet 1990;i:1280.
19. Durand E, LeJeunne C, Hugues FC. Failure of prophylactic zidovudine after suicidal self-inoculation of HIV-infected blood. N Engl J Med 1991;324:1062.
20. Lafon SW, Mooney BD, McMullen JP, Pattishall KH, Smiley ML, Rogers MD, Lehrman SN. A double-blind, placebo-controlled study of the safety of Retrovir (Zidovudine, ZDV). Interscience Conference on Antimicrobial Agents and Chemotherapy, Atlanta, Georgia, 1990:167 (abstr. 489).

Glossary

Acquired immunodeficiency syndrome (AIDS). A set of serious clinical ailments resulting from severe immune dysfunction caused by infection with the human immunodeficiency virus (HIV).

Adult T-cell leukemia/lymphoma (ATLL). A malignant proliferation mature T-cells associated with infiltrative lesions of the skin and viscera, lytic bone lesions, and hypercalcemia.

Antibody. A complex set of proteins (immunoglobulins) found in the blood and produced by the B cells in response to exposure to specific foreign molecules or antigens. Antibodies have the ability to combine with the specific antigen that stimulated antibody production. At present, five classes of antibodies are distinguishable: immunoglobulins G (IgG), M (IgM), A (IgA), D (IgD), and E (IgE). Antibodies can neutralize toxins and interact with various elements of the immune system to eliminate infectious organisms from the body.

Antigen. A substance that, when introduced into the body of a human or other animal, stimulates the production of antibodies that react specifically with that antigen.

AIDS-related complex (ARC). A assortment of chronic symptoms and physical findings that are found in persons infected with HIV but do not meet the Centers for Disease Control definition of AIDS. Included in the symptoms are lymphadenopathy, chronic diarrhea, unintentional weight loss, lethargy, recurrent fevers, oral thrush, and certain changes in the patient's immune system. ARC may or may not develop into AIDS. ARC is an outdated term and is rarely used anymore.

Autoradiography. Production of an image on an x-ray film by a radioactively labeled substance.

B Lymphocyte (or B cell). A type of white blood cell that produces antibody in response to stimulation initiated by an antigen.

CD4 lymphocyte or T4 cell. A T lymphocyte that expresses the cell-surface marker molecule CD4. These cells are believed to consist mainly of helper/inducer lymphocytes, which secrete many soluble molecules and play a significant role in the regulation of the human immune system. These cells are the main target for infection with HIV.

CD8 lymphocyte or CD8 T cell. A T lymphocyte that expresses the cell-surface marker molecule CD8. These cells are believed to mainly consist of suppressor/cytotoxic lymphocytes, which play significant functional and regulatory roles in the human immune system.

Cell-mediated immunity. A defense mechanism of the immune system involving the coordinated activity of at least two groups of T lymphocytes, namely, helper T cells and killer T cells. The helper produces various substances that regulate and stimulate other cellular components of the immune system. The role of the killer T lymphocyte is to destroy cells in the body bearing foreign antigens (e.g., cells infected with viruses).

Chromosome. A rodlike structure found in the cell nucleus that contains the genes of that cell. Chromosomes are composed of DNA and proteins. They can be seen under the light microscope during certain stages of cell division.

Core antigens. Protein antigens that constitute the internal structure or core of the virus.

Cytomegalovirus (CMV). A member of the herpesvirus group of viruses that rarely causes disease in healthy adults. CMV is known to cause a severe congenital infection of infants and life-threatening infections in patients requiring immune suppression. In AIDS patients, however, CMV may result in pneumonia and inflammation of the retina, liver, colon, and kidney.

Cytopathic. Ability to induce pathologic changes to cells.

DNA (deoxyribonucleic acid). The substance of heredity. The large nucleic acid found mainly in the chromosomes of the nucleus of living cells, responsible for transmitting hereditary characteristics of an organism. DNA is composed of the sugar deoxyribose, phosphate, and the bases adenine, thymine, guanine, and cytosine.

DNA denaturation. The separation of DNA into its two strands of polynucleotides, e.g., by exposing it to near-boiling temperatures.

DNA probe. A specific sequence of single-stranded DNA (ssDNA) used to seek out a complementary sequence in other single strands of DNA or RNA. The probe is usually tagged with either a radioactive molecule or various nonradioactive molecules so that it can be detected.

DNA sequencing. The process of determining the nucleotide sequence of DNA.

EIA or ELISA. Acronyms for "enzyme immunoassay" or "enzyme-linked immunosorbent assay", respectively. The terms are used interchangeably and represent a test used to detect antibodies against HIV in blood samples. It is an assay based on antigen–antibody interactions, which uses enzymes attached to an antibody to measure the reaction.

Electrophoresis. A method of separating molecules, such as DNA fragments or proteins, by using an electric field to make them move through a medium, such as agarose or polyacrylamide gel, at rates that correspond to their electric charge and size.

Encephalitis. An inflammation of the brain.

Encephalopathy. Any of a variety of degenerative diseases of the brain.

***env*.** Represents the gene for or the structural proteins of the envelope of retroviruses.

Envelope antigens. Proteins that comprise the envelope or surface of a virus.

Epstein–Barr virus (EBV). A member of the herpesvirus family of viruses. It is believed to be the etiologic agent of mononucleosis in young adults and has been implicated in the development of Burkitt's lymphoma in Africa.

False-negative. A negative test result for a sample from a person who is truly positive for the condition. The patient is incorrectly diagnosed as not having a particular disease or characteristic.

False-positive. A positive test result for a sample from a person who is truly negative for the condition. The person is incorrectly diagnosed as having a particular disease or characteristic.

***gag*.** Literally means group-specific antigen. Represents the gene for the structural proteins of the core of retroviruses.

Gene. A unit of heredity; a segment of the DNA molecule containing the code for a specific function.

Gene expression. The manifestation of the genetic material of an organism as specific traits. Specific gene products are expressed as proteins.

Genome. The full genetic or gene complement of an organism.

Gold standard. In biomedical testing, it is the independent test that unequivocaly verifies the presence or absence of the condition being tested for.

Hemophilia. A hereditary bleeding disorder of males, inherited through the mother and caused by a deficiency in the ability to make one or more blood-clotting factors.

Herpes simplex. Acute diseases caused by the herpes simplex viruses types 1 and 2. Painful blisters form on the skin and mucous membranes, especially on the borders of the lip (type 1) or the mucous surface of the genitals.

Herpesviruses group. A group of large DNA-containing viruses that includes the herpes simplex viruses, the varicella-zoster virus (etiologic agent of chickenpox and shingles), cytomegalovirus, and Epstein–Barr virus.

HIV (human immunodeficiency virus). The name selected by the International Committee on the Taxonomy of Viruses for the etiologic agent of AIDS (originally termed HTLV-III, LAV, or ARV). HIV is a member of the retrovirus family of viruses.

Human T-lymphotropic virus type I (HTLV-I). The first known human retrovirus and is unrelated to HIV. It infects T-lymphocytes and is associated etiologically with adult T-cell leukemia/lymphoma (ATLL) and tropical spastic paraperesis (TSP) also known as HTV-I associated myelopathy (HAM).

Human T-lymphotropic virus type II (HTLV-II). The second human retrovirus to be identified. HTLV-II is very similar to HTLV-I and there is extensive serological cross-reactivity between proteins of the two viruses. HTLV-II is currently a virus in search of a disease.

Humoral immunity. The part of the human immune defense mechanism that involves the production of antibodies and associated components, present mainly in body fluids such as serum and lymph.

Hybridization. The coming together of single strands on nucleic acids so that they adhere (by hydrogen bonding) and form a double strand. The technique of hybridization is used in conjunction with probes to detect the presence or absence of specific complementary sequences of nucleic acids.

Immune system. The system of defense mechanisms of the body, in which specialized cells and proteins (including antibodies) in the blood and other body fluids work together to eliminate disease-producing microorganisms and other foreign substances.

Immunoglobulin. A group of serum proteins with antibody activity.

Indirect immunofluorescence assay (IFA). An assay based on the detection of antigen–antibody interactions (the antigen is expressed on an infected cell) using a second antibody tagged with fluorescent compound (e.g., fluorescein).

Interferons. A class of proteins involved in immune function and containing inhibitory capability for certain viral infections.

Interleukin-2 (IL-2). A substance produced by T lymphocytes capable of stimulating activated T lymphocytes and possibly selected B lymphocytes to proliferate.

In vitro. Refers to those experiments conducted in an artificial environment such as in tissue culture.

In vivo. Refers to those experiments conducted in living animals or humans.

Interstitial pneumonia. Localized acute inflammation of the lung.

Kaposi's sarcoma. A tumor or cancer of the blood or lymphatic vessel walls. It generally appears as blue-violet to brownish skin blotches or bumps. AIDS-associated Kaposi's sarcoma is much more aggressive than the earlier, more rare form of the disease found in the United States and Europe, where it occurs primarily in men over aged 50 to 60 years, usually those of Mediterranean origin.

Lentiviruses. A subfamily of retroviruses that includes HIV. These viruses produce diverse chronic diseases in their host. They produce an acute cytocidal infection followed by a slowly developing multisystem disease including encephalitis. Associated with this process is a persistent virus infection and the development of viral latency following the initial viremic phase.

Lymphocyte. A white blood cell that is part of the immune system.

Macrophage. A form of white blood cell that has the ability to ingest or phagocytize foreign particulate matter, such as bacteria. Macrophages have the further job of presenting foreign antigen to the appropriate lymphocyte subgroup and thereby activating it.

Messenger RNA (mRNA). A RNA copy of the genetic information contained in DNA and used to direct the synthesis of specific proteins outside the nucleus.

Mitogen. A substance that induces cell division.

Monoclonal antibodies (MAb). Antibodies derived from a single-cell clone of antibody cells. MAbs are a homogeneous population of antibodies that recognize only one type of antigen.

Monocyte. A phagocytic white blood cell that develops into a macrophage and engulfs and destroys bacterial and other disease-causing microorganisms.

Mycobacterium avium-intracellulare. A bacterium, related to the organism that causes tuberculosis in humans, which rarely caused disease in man before AIDS.

Nucleic acids. DNA and RNA, the molecules that carry genetic information.

Nucleotides. A building block of DNA or RNA. It is composed of one base, one phosphate, and one sugar molecule (deoxyribose in DNA, ribose in RNA).

Oligonucleotide. A short string of nucleotides.

Oligonucleotide probe. A short DNA sequence synthesized from a known gene sequence.

Peripheral blood mononuclear cells (PBMCs). A group of white blood cells found in the peripheral blood compartment consisting of monocytes, large granular lymphocytes, B-cells, and T-cells.

Persistent generalized lymphadenopathy (PGL). A condition characterized by persistent, generalized swollen lymph glands.

Phagocyte. A blood or tissue cell that binds to, engulfs, and destroys microorganisms, damaged cells, and foreign particles.

Pneumocystis carinii pneumonia. A pneumonia that is caused by the parasite *Pneumocystis carinii* and is the most common life-threatening opportunistic infection diagnosed in AIDS patients.

Pol. The polymerase gene of retroviruses.

Polymerase chain reaction (PCR). A technique originally developed for the selective in vitro enzymatic amplification of targeted DNA sequences up to 10^6 times or more.

polymorphism. A single gene trait that exists in two or more alternative forms (e.g., HLA class II antigen).

Predictive value. The proportion of persons with positive test results that have the condition being tested for.

Provirus. A DNA copy of the genetic information of a retrovirus that can be integrated into the DNA of the infected cell. Copies of the provirus are passed on to each of the infected cell's daughter cells.

Radioimmunoprecipitation assay (RIPA). An assay based on precipitation of an antigen–antibody. One component of the complex, usually the antigen, is radioactive so as to be able to measure the precipitated complex.

Restriction enzyme (or restriction endonuclease). An enzyme that recognizes a specific nucleotide sequence (usually four to six nucleotides) in double-stranded DNA. The enzyme cuts both strands of the DNA molecule at every place where this sequence appears.

Retrovirus. A family of viruses that contain their genetic information in the form of RNA and that have the ability to copy the RNA into DNA (using the viral enzyme reverse transcriptase) inside an infected cell. The resulting DNA is incorporated into the genetic structure of the cell in the form of a provirus.

Reverse transcriptase (RT). An enzyme possessed by all retroviruses that allows them to produce a DNA copy (provirus) of their RNA genetic information. This is an early step in the virus's natural life cycle.

RNA (ribonucleic acid). The ribose-containing nucleic acid associated with the control of chemical activities inside a cell. It can also be the form in which various viruses contain their genetic information.

SDS-PAGE (sodium dodecyl sulfate-polyacrylamide gel electrophoresis). A technique for the separation of molecules (principally proteins) by the differential migration through a gel (composed of a polymer of acrylamide termed, polyacrylamide) according to the size of the molecules in an electrical field.

Sensitivity. In serologic testing, the percentage of people who test positive in a particular test and who in fact do have the condition being tested for.

Seroconversion. The initial development of detectable antibodies specific to a particular antigan.

Seropositive. The condition in which antibodies to a specific antigen, such as antibodies to HIV, are found in the blood.

Specificity. In serologic testing, the percentage of people who test negative in a particular test and who in fact do not have the condition being tested for.

SIV (simian immunodeficiency virus). A virus of subhuman primates (e.g., sooty mangabey monkeys) that can cause immunodeficiency and AIDS, and which is closely related the human immunodeficiency virus type 2 (HIV-2).

Tropical spastic paraperesis (TSP). A degenerative neurological disease characterized by weakness in the lower extremities, sensory disturbances, and urinary incontinence.

T4/T8 cell ratios. The ratio of T4 cells (helper cells) to T8 cels (suppressor cells). Persons with AIDS have a deficiency of T4 cells and a low ratio of T4 to T8 cells.

T lymphocyte (or T cell). A cell that matures in the thymus gland. These cells are found primarily in the blood, lymph, and lymphoid organs. Subsets of T cells have a wide variety of specialized functions within the immune system.

T4 lymphocyte (or T4 cell). A synonym for CD4 T helper/inducer cell.

T8 lymphocyte (or T8 cell). A synonym for CD8 T suppressor cell.

Viremia. The presence of virus in circulating blood, which implies active viral replication.

Virion. A complete virus particle.

Western blot (WB). A test that involves the identification of a person's antibodies against specific proteins of the virus. Western blot is at least as specific as the EIA test and is the confirmatory test most widely used on samples found to be repeatedly reactive on EIA tests.

Zidovudine (AZT). The HIV reverse transcriptase inhibitor 3′-azido-3′-deoxythymidine that is licensed by the U.S. Food and Drug Administration for the treatment of HIV infection and AIDS. The drug is known to inhibit the multiplication of HIV.

Index

N

O

P

Q